# Clinical Tropical Medicine

VOLUME II

**Malaria**
**Amebiasis**
**Cholera**

*Edited by*

KEVIN M. CAHILL, M.D., D.T.M. & H. (LOND.)

*Director, The Tropical Disease Center*
*St. Clare's Hospital*
*New York*

*and*

*Professor of Tropical Medicine*
*The Royal College of Surgeons in Ireland*
*Dublin*

## University Park Press

*BALTIMORE • LONDON • TOKYO*

*Published 1972 by University Park Press*
*Chamber of Commerce Building*
*Baltimore, Maryland 21202*

*Copyright © 1972 New York Academy of Medicine*
*Library of Congress Catalog Card No. 70-38920*
*ISBN No. 0-8391-0501-0*

Printed in U.S.A.

# Clinical Tropical Medicine

*Previous books by Kevin M. Cahill, M.D.*

TROPICAL DISEASES IN TEMPERATE CLIMATES
HEALTH ON THE HORN OF AFRICA
THE UNTAPPED RESOURCE: MEDICINE AND DIPLOMACY
MEDICAL ADVICE FOR THE TRAVELER
CLINICAL TROPICAL MEDICINE — VOLUME I

For Helen and Hugh

# CONTRIBUTORS

John D. Arnold, M.D.

*Professor of Medicine, University of Missouri, Kansas City, Mo.*

Abram S. Benenson, M.D.

*Professor of Community Medicine, University of Kentucky, Lexington, Ky.*

Leonard J. Bruce-Chwatt, M.D.

*Professor of Tropical Hygiene and Director, The Ross Institute, London School of Hygiene and Tropical Medicine, London, England*

Kevin M. Cahill, M.D.

*Director, The Tropical Disease Center, St. Clare's Hospital, New York, and Professor of Tropical Medicine, The Royal College of Surgeons in Ireland, Dublin*

Craig J. Canfield, M.D.

*Chief, Clinical Malaria Unit, Walter Reed Army Institute of Research, Washington, D.C.*

Charles J. Carpenter, M.D.

*Professor of Medicine, The Johns Hopkins Medical School, Baltimore, Md.*

Peter G. Contacos, M.D.

*Head, Section on Primate Malaria, National Institutes of Allergy and Infectious Diseases, Atlanta, Ga.*

John Duffy, Ph.D.

*Professor of the History of Medicine, Tulane University Medical School, New Orleans, La.*

Ronald Elsdon-Dew, M.D.

*Director, Amebiasis Research Unit, Durban, South Africa*

George U. Fisher, M.D.

*Malaria Surveillance Officer, National Communicable Disease Center, Atlanta, Ga.*

Eugene J. Gangarosa, M.D.

*Deputy Chief, Bacterial Disease Branch, National Center for Disease Control, U.S.P.H.S., Atlanta, Ga.*

George R. Healy, Ph.D.

*Chief, Helminthology and Protozoology Unit, National Center for Disease Control, Atlanta, Ga.*

Victor G. Heiser, M.D.

*Former Director of the Far East, Rockefeller Foundation, New York*

Thomas R. Hendrix, M.D.

*Professor of Medicine, The Johns Hopkins Medical School, Baltimore, Md.*

Robert B. Hornick, M.D.

*Professor of Medicine, University of Maryland School of Medicine, Baltimore, Md.*

Kerrison Juniper, M.D.

*Professor of Medicine, University of Arkansas Medical School, Little Rock, Ark.*

Irvin G. Kagan, Ph.D.

*Chief, Parasitology Section, National Center for Disease Control, U.S.P.H.S., Atlanta, Ga.*

Brian Maegraith, M.D.

*Dean, The Liverpool School of Tropical Medicine, Liverpool, England*

Harry Most, M.D.

*Professor of Preventive Medicine, New York University School of Medicine, New York*

R. A. Neal, Ph.D.

*Director, The Wellcome Laboratories of Tropical Medicine, England*

S. John Powell, M.D.

*Professor of Medicine, University of Natal, Durban, South Africa*

Paul F. Russell, M.D.

*Staff Member Emeritus, The Rockefeller Foundation, New York*

# CONTENTS

# Cholera

# PREFACE

This volume is another collection of three in the series of Symposia in Clinical Tropical Medicine. The approach to, goals of, and acknowledgements for this series were clearly stated in the Preface to Volume I and apply here in equal measure:

> These programs have been planned on the premise that tropical medicine is a clinical field of great significance to the American physician today. For too many years tropical medicine in this country has been relegated to the parasitology laboratories, and taught as an esoteric topic representing the final preclinical hurdle for the medical student. This view, always unfortunate, is no longer tenable in the United States. As the leader of the free world our overseas commitments are vast, and it seems to me, they involve, as a primary objective, the welfare of peoples in the developing nations of the world.
>
> The costs of these symposia were partially funded by a generous grant from the Merck Company Foundation. They have all been published in the *Bulletin of the New York Academy of Medicine* and a deep debt of gratitude is due to the Editor, Dr. Saul Jarcho and the Associate Editor, Mr. Franklin Furness, for their continued interest in tropical medicine as well as for their superb editing.
>
> This series will continue and other volumes will follow. Throughout these symposia I have attempted to select topics and data of relevance to the clinician in the U.S.A. as well as in the tropics, and to present them in an orderly but exciting fashion; this approach will be maintained. It is my hope that the presentations on schistosomiasis and hepatitis, balanced by a description of the contributions of our predecessors in tropical medicine, will serve not only the immediate needs of health workers concerned with these infections, but will stimulate them and others to further research in the field of clinical tropical medicine.

The three "tropical" infections considered in this book are currently of major interest to physicians and other medical workers in the temperate as well as the torrid zones. In the United States, for example, the incidence of malaria increased by more than twenty times in the last five years. This infection must now be considered in the differential diagnosis of fevers not only in

Vietnam veterans and other travelers, but in blood transfusion recipients, and drug addicts, and in many states where indigenous mosquito transmission of malaria can and has occurred. The world-wide incidence of amebiasis is detailed in this text, but the frequency of clinically recognized cases in this country is related more to the index of suspicion of the good clinician in a community than to the percentage of the population harboring *E. histolytica.* Cholera, as I note in the introduction to that section, epitomizes the "tropical" infection in this jet age, moving from a localized endemic disease to its present status as a health challenge around the world.

One symposium in this series has been separately published.[1] In that book the relationship of medicine and diplomacy was considered by an unusually qualified group of experts including the President of the United Nations and representatives from the disciplines of diplomacy, economics and legislature, as well as voluntary agencies and tropical medicine. The philosophy of that book was translated into a specific bill for America, "The International Health Agency Act of 1971," by one of its contributors, Congressman Hugh L. Carey. For his services to tropical medicine, and for the great good and joy that both he and his fine wife have brought to this earth I dedicate this volume.

KMC

---

1. Cahill, K., *The Untapped Resource* — Medicine and Diplomacy, Orbis Press, Maryknoll, N.Y., 115 pp., 1971.

# SYMPOSIUM ON MALARIA

## Introduction*

### Kevin M. Cahill

Director, Tropical Disease Center
St. Clare's Hospital and Health Center
New York, N. Y.

Professor of Tropical Medicine
Royal College of Surgeons
Dublin, Ireland

MALARIA, as on innumerable occasions in history, is at present re-emerging as an unconquered foe of primary importance to physicians, politicians, soldiers, generals, and persons of *all* levels in *all* nations of the world. The impact of resistant malaria affects America, for example, not merely in the highlands of Vietnam, where more troops are invalided by plasmodia than by battle wounds, but in this country where relapses are occurring increasingly after a victim's discharge from the armed forces.

This has posed new and urgent challenges for civilian clinicians, public health workers, laboratory technicians, blood-bank directors, and many others across the land. An ever-growing number of tourists and businessmen are traveling from the United States to malarious areas, and the physician of 1969 must be able not only to advise his

*Presented as part of a *Symposium on Malaria* held by The Tropical Disease Center, St. Clare's Hospital, New York, N. Y., and The Merck Company Foundation, Rahway, N. J., at the Center May 17, 1969.

patient on antimalarial prophylaxis but must be attuned to the possibility of malaria in its myriad clinical patterns.

For this fourth in the series of *Symposia in Clinical Tropical Medicine* we are exceedingly fortunate that distinguished malariologists have been able to come from many areas and busy schedules to participate. L. J. Bruce-Chwatt was chief of the malaria research and development section of the World Health Organization before assuming his new position as director of the Ross Institute in London, England. His philosophic and historic review of *Malaria Eradication at the Crossroads* is therefore a uniquely informed presentation of a crucial decision that will affect future generations of mankind. Paul Russell, this country's senior malariologist, comments succinctly and perceptively on Dr. Bruce-Chwatt's paper. George Fisher's epidemiologic analysis of malaria in the United States details the problem here, while Irving Kagan's comprehensive survey of serologic tests to ease the diagnosis of malaria adumbrates a feasible approach for laboratories in the future.

The clinical complications of malaria are presented by three leading experts: Brian Maegraith from Liverpool, England, and Harry Most and Craig Canfield of this country. The present prophylactic and therapeutic approaches to malaria are detailed by John Arnold and Peter G. Contacos. Most of these men then contribute their experience and thoughts to a wide-ranging discussion of particular problems in the clinical management of a disease that has been a scourge since the dawn of mankind, is intertwined with the history of nations, with the rise and fall of civilizations, and is with us again as a significant medical problem in America today.

# MALARIA ERADICATION AT THE CROSSROADS*

LEONARD J. BRUCE-CHWATT

Professor of Tropical Hygiene
London School of Hygiene and Tropical Medicine
London, England

A MONG the endemic diseases whose burdens fall on the developing countries of the world malaria holds one of the first places.

The *Third Report on the World Health Situation*[19] indicates that malaria is one of the 10 most important health problems of the 90 countries that reported. In the African Region 14 of 20 countries reported malaria as their major health problem. This was also the conclusion of the report on tropical health prepared by the National Academy of Sciences in Washington, D.C.[1]

The global program of eradicating malaria stimulated and coordinated by WHO and so generously assisted by the United States is now in its 13th year. How far have we progressed in eliminating malaria from the world? How far are we still from this goal?

A brief description of a program of this size can be given only in broadest lines, like those of an artist's sketch of a "landscape with figures." Some of the figures that stand out in such a landscape are revealing. The numerical figures of the achievements and perspectives of malaria eradication are significant, as they indicate not only what has been accomplished but also what remains to be done. As usual with such data it is easier to measure something than to know exactly what is being measured.

The latest report of WHO submitted in May 1968 to the World Health Assembly[2] indicates that out of 1,716 million people living in malarious or previously malarious areas (without counting mainland China, North Korea, and North Vietnam, which do not submit any reports to WHO) eradication programs are virtually completed in countries or territories inhabited by 648 million people; these programs are well advanced over areas inhabited by 711 million. Thus 1,359 million or

*Presented as part of a *Symposium on Malaria* sponsored by The Tropical Disease Center, St. Clare's Hospital, New York, N.Y. and The Merck Company Foundation, Rahway, N.J., held at the Center, May 17, 1969.

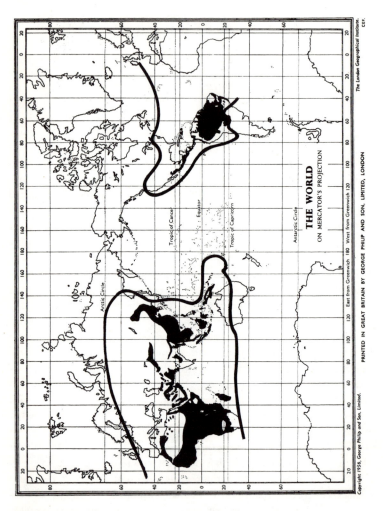

Global past and present extension of malaria. The line represents the original extent of malarious areas of the world. Areas where endemic malaria transmission still occurred in 1968 are shown in black. Reproduced by permission of the publisher.

79% of people living in malarious areas are enjoying completely or partially the benefits conferred by eradication activities.

Malaria has been eliminated from the whole of Europe, from the Asian part of the Soviet Union, from Israel, Lebanon, Syria, and some neighboring countries of the Middle East, from large parts of India and Ceylon, from Japan, from most of North America including the whole of the United States, from several islands in the Caribbean, from nearly the whole territory of Venezuela and much of the southern portion of South America, from the southern tip of Africa, from Mauritius, from the northern part of Australia, and from Taiwan. The eradication program has been completed in 36 of the 146 countries or territories where malaria was originally present.

It is estimated that over the past decade deaths due to malaria decreased from 2.5 million every year to well below one million. Even more important is the fact that the over-all annual morbidity due to malaria has decreased from 250 million cases to about 50 million. Such a striking decrease of sickness and death must have produced immense gains in health and fitness on a world scale.

However in countries inhabited by 364 million people eradication programs are either in an early stage or have not yet materialized. This figure for the most part represents the countries of Africa, but it also includes many countries of the Far East and of South America. About half of this population inhabits 21 countries where preeradication programs are now in operation or are about to begin, but their effect on the incidence of malaria has been slight.

If we judge our achievements by what has been done the results are excellent, but if we calculate the distance that remains before we reach the goal of eradicating malaria from the globe, it appears that the remaining one quarter of our unfinished task will probably be more difficult than all that we have done before.

There is no denying that during the past three years the global program has slowed down and that there have been some serious reverses.

In Ceylon, where two years ago the major part of the country, which had 12 million people, was in the consolidation phase of malaria eradication, an epidemic of vivax malaria with more than 1 million cases occurred in 1967-1968. In the gigantic program for India, with 500 million people (of whom well over one half live in areas in the maintenance phase), the incidence of malaria increased in the north and central provinces, and it has been necessary to reinstitute spraying with insecticides to deal with focal outbreaks and to prevent further deterioration. In Pakistan, as in India, the extension of effective antimalaria activities in large urban zones has met with serious obstacles and Karachi became a malarious island within a largely nonmalarious rural area. There has been an outbreak of malaria in Paraguay, where 50,000 cases were reported.

Even during the early years of the global program certain difficulties of malaria eradication became obvious in a few areas. The nature of these difficulties has been assessed by the World Health Organization,[3-8] the means needed to overcome the obstacles have been outlined, and appropriate action has been taken whenever possible. In spite of the existence of some "problem areas" the progress in eradicating malaria has been satisfactory in terms of the steady extension of areas in the "consolidation" or "maintenance" phases of the program. However the hard core of endemic areas inhabited by 300 to 400 million people in the tropics has remained static over the past decade in spite of a score of pilot projects that were carried out, generally with little success. A few successful pilot projects in which malaria transmission was interrupted created a paradoxical situation. In spite of these single successes the implementation of a program for eradicating malaria was impossible because of the shortages of basic health services and administrative or financial obstacles that made the final achievement of a countrywide program unlikely. Moreover a program limited to one country surrounded by others where the eradication of malaria was not contemplated created additional risks due to the notorious and always underestimated mobility of human populations.

It is true that some countries adopted the concept of eradication too hastily, without the necessary planning or resources and without providing for the necessary basic health services which would eventually undertake much of the case detection activities in the final phases of malaria eradication.

The need of such services has been recognized, and since 1960 about 20 "preeradication programs" have been developed with the main objective of gradually building up the necessary facilities and especially the rural health services and the training of auxiliary personnel. However the progress of preeradication programs has been slow because of the shortage of suitable man power and lack of funds.

From the early days of malaria eradication there have been two schools of thought with different views on the relation between health and socioeconomic advance.

One school believed that the eradication of malaria—or any other major endemic disease—leads not only to greater individual health but provides an effective lever for economic and social advance which cannot proceed unless the burden of sickness is lifted to give men the strength and the desire to build a better life for themselves.

The other school felt that the satisfactory completion and maintenance of a program for eradicating malaria depends on an adequate socioeconomic level of the country and that without it no permanent success can be expected.

The role of malaria eradication as a spearhead for economic development in areas where the disease interfered with the expansion of agriculture or industry has been sufficiently underlined by Pampana.[15]

More recently MacKenzie[16] in describing the eradication program in Thailand pointed out that even apparently costly antimalaria measures are cheap in relation to long-term benefits that they bring, by making the transmission of the infection only a marginal risk and increasing the productive output of rural communities.

Without attempting to disparage the essential truth of the statement that the rapid progress of any country can be seriously hampered by the widespread illness of its population, the present consensus on eradicating malaria in developing countries maintains that the final outcome of such a campaign may be compromised by a lack of adequate administrative organization and basic health services.

The problem has been widely discussed by Gonzales[9] in the context of mass campaigns and general health services, and his conclusion was that the two approaches are not mutually exclusive, though their progressive convergence depends on a number of factors, and that the realistic planning of such a combined strategy demands a careful assessment of human and financial resources.

During the first years of eradicating malaria from the globe the main emphasis was laid on the high technical standards of the methods of attack; problems related to socioeconomic conditions of the counties concerned or to many sided aspects of human ecology were certainly recognized but their full relevance became more obvious only gradually.

7

Realistic assessment of the difficulties that have slowed down the previous striking advance of programs for eradicating malaria have now stressed the importance of all the administrative, socioeconomic, financial, and political problems that form part of the enormous and unsolved dilemma of bringing the underdeveloped part of the world to the level of the more advanced countries.

It appears that the forthcoming reassessment of the strategy of WHO in eradicating malaria will be related to three important factors: the impact of malaria on socioeconomic development; the cost of malaria eradication in relation to the material and man-power resources of some countries; and the difficulty of achieving eradication with deficient basic health services and increased mobility of the population.

It is difficult to predict the changes that may be introduced into the present strategy, as this depends on the findings of consultative groups requested to provide factual data, especially on programs that have made good initial progress and are unable to complete the task according to the original plan.

It is likely however that every effort will be made without too much delay to assist those countries where the eradication of malaria has reasonable chances of success.

When it comes to countries where the shortage of human and material resources does not indicate the early possibility of completing a program for the eradication of malaria, which depends so much on near-perfect methodology and on an all-out effort, a reversion to activities of malaria control should not be regarded as a defeat. During this temporary stage the improvement of basic health services may prepare the ground for a future successful program.

The accelerated training of medical and auxiliary staff is certainly the most urgent task for the next decades. This training should be adapted to the immediate needs of the countries concerned and should have a strong bias in favor of preventive medicine.

The reasons for the priority of medical training in any health plan for developing countries of Africa are generally known, but some recent figures will throw a sharper light on the situation. Twenty-six countries of tropical Africa had a total of 4,700 fully qualified doctors in 1962, or 1 doctor per 18,000. In 1965 the number was 4,400 and the relevant proportion was 1 doctor to 20,500. The loss was largely due to the departure of expatriate doctors and to the immigration of African physicians to countries where the financial rewards are better. This outflow of trained personnel from Africa is one of the paradoxes of our time. In the 11 medical schools now existing in Africa the annual output is about 170 newly trained doctors; by 1970 this figure should reach 400. But the population of 200 million of the African region is now increasing by about 4 million every year and if the minimal ratio of 1 doctor to 10,000 people is to be reached, then 400 new graduates are required annually to keep pace only with the normal increase of the population, and any improvement of the situation will still be distant.

There can be no permanent improvement of the present conditions of health in developing countries generally and those of tropical Africa in particular unless the highest possible priority is given to the training of adequate numbers of fully qualified health workers: doctors, nurses, midwives, laboratory technicians, sanitarians and, last but not least, efficient medical administrators. The response to this challenge will determine the future of the world's health in this century.

Diseases of the tropics are becoming increasingly common in countries situated in temperate climates. There is no absolute safety from any infection as long as vast reservoirs of pathogens are present in some areas of the globe. The speed and volume of human mobility today can be judged by the fact that in 1966 there were about 120 million international and intercontinental travelers of whom one third made the journey by air. This figure, probably underestimated, is expected to increase by about 8% every year. The London Airport at Heathrow handled during the past year about 15 million passengers and, with the arrival of superjets it is predicted that the airport will be coping with 20 million passengers in 1971 and with 24 million in 1973.

Each of the Boeing 747 planes can carry 390 to 500 passengers, and it is estimated that at peak times three of these "human containers" will be landing within half an hour. This will mean that almost 2,400 people will pass through the airport building after completion of the passport and health formalities.

The danger of the importation of exotic disease into countries with a temperate climate has been stressed by Maegraith,[10, 11] and Dorolle[12] has recently pointed out the increasing importance for international health of the phenomenon of mass travel.

P. N. Dorolle, deputy director-general of WHO, advocated an international approach to the problem of combating disease before it enters a country and pointed out the need of keeping track of travellers in case they develop symptoms. "In this age of jet planes and soon of supersonic transport the only way of preventing the old plagues, and some new ones, from spreading from country to country is to help the poorest nations in the world to reach such a level of economic and technical development that it will be possible for them to combat the evil at its source."

Although the spread of imported malaria is not very likely in North America or Europe there is little doubt that undiagnosed cases of this infection will claim more victims. Moreover the massive introduction of carriers into countries where the eradication of malaria is in one of the final phases may seriously endanger the outcome of the national program.

The difficulties of some malaria eradication programs were classified as administrative and socioeconomic, and as technical. The second group, of technical obstacles, stimulated a great deal of research, much of which was assisted by WHO,[13] although the more recent program of research on malaria sponsored by the U.S. Army dwarfs by its scope and means any other coordinated scheme of this kind.[14]

During the past decade various lines of research on malaria received different emphasis, and this was related to the gradual building up and progress of global eradication of malaria. Early interests were concentrated on the technical problems of application of residual insecticides, on the development of various formulations suitable for sorptive surfaces, on assessment of the duration of activity of the insecticidal deposits, and on the development of suitable spraying equipment. Later the appearance of resistance to insecticides led to the development of techniques for assessing the susceptibility of vectors, to studies of the dynamics of this phenomenon, and to the synthesis, screening, and field trials of new insecticides.

The problem of resistance of malaria parasites to reliable drugs opened wide areas for multidisciplinary research ranging from biochemistry of the parasite at the cell level to development of injectable repository drugs and large-scale laboratory screening of various compounds.

More recent studies comprise the dynamics of transmitting malaria, the study of the epidemiology of disappearing disease, *in vitro* culture of plasmodia, development of new immunological techniques for the case detection or prevention of disease, and investigation of the relation between human and simian malaria.

Many other studies too numerous to mention have shown that all types of research are interdependent and that at times a fundamental approach may help in solving a practical problem. On the other hand some field observations followed up experimentally may give rise to the development of a branch of basic science.

The future development of research in malaria will depend on the speed with which the goal of global eradication can be approached. Experience has shown that in spite of the advent of residual insecticides and synthetic antimalarials, the effective methods of using these weapons are often too expensive for the limited resources of developing countries. The eradication of malaria has been achieved in many large areas of the world, but unless the methodology is further simplified eradication of malaria from the globe, though theoretically possible, will continue to be unattainable for many years to come. Simpler methods of breaking the malaria cycle of transmission will have to be found through intensive research on vector and parasite biology, insecticides, chemotherapy, and immunology.

Studies of the biochemical mechanisms and genetics of resistance of malaria to insecticides should help with the appraisal of new potent and safe imagicides and larvicides. Intensive research on biological methods of vector control will continue in response to the demand for integrated procedures.

The resistance of some strains of malaria parasites to drugs may assume greater importance in limited areas of the world, and investigations on the spectrum and dynamics of drug-fastness are bound to come to the fore. It is to be hoped that research on the chemotherapy of malaria will be expanded and based on firmer biochemical foundations than heretofore. Studies on malaria in animals will be of great value in this respect and appropriate screening methods are bound to improve the final assessment of new compounds, although trials of drugs on natural or induced cases of human malaria will always be the final criterion of the value of a new compound and of its toxicity to man.

Much attention will need to be paid to the epidemiological approach in planning eradication programs so that they will be closely related to basic public health services. More emphasis should be given to the improvement of epidemiological methodology in the late phases of

11

eradication. This calls for better case detection, perhaps by new protozoological, immunological, or electronic methods.

Better knowledge of human ecology is needed to improve the methods of health education and to adapt them to various cultural patterns. Experience has shown that most of the operations of attack can be carried out provided there are good public relations. In the consolidation phase of eradicating malaria, when the annual incidence of malaria is less than 100 cases per 1 million of population, the urge to eradicate the infection decreases rapidly. Much remains to be done to convince populations and their authorities that unless the programs continue much of the benefit will be lost. Studies on socioeconomic advantages of control and eradication of malaria may provide better guidance of medical administrators.

The timing of integration of eradicating malaria into general health services, the transformation of the organization of the eradication of malaria into a multipurpose health organization, and the training arrangements for the various activities should be given special attention in operational research.

Over the past decade the gradual recognition of gaps in our knowledge have led to the increased emphasis on a greater scientific effort to find new means for the attack on the parasite and its vector. However the present gratifying faith in research and support of it may lead to disappointments if the scientist is expected to overcome all or most of the obstacles that slow down the progress of eradicating malaria.

Medical advances do not arise in a social vacuum. They are products of the scientific knowledge of the time and of the demands of the community. Medicine is an aspect of social technology, but its goals and ethics are the products of the interplay between scientific understanding and human aspirations.

Although a concentrated scientific effort may create new methods of potential value to preventive medicine the timely and proper use of these means depends on the society, which must have the will, the resources, and the favorable environment to apply the existing knowledge to the promotion of health.

There is little doubt that successful antimalaria measures play an important part in reducing mortality and morbidity and that in this way they increase the length of life. No wonder that the malarialogists have often been called "sorcerer's apprentices" unable to control the demo-

12

graphic forces that they apparently unleash by contributing to a "population explosion" in developing countries. One wonders if this accusation is fair on a global scale even if it may be true in some rather exceptional areas.

During the past decade the fatality rate due to malaria was estimated at 1% and the number of deaths attributable to this disease decreased from 2.5 million to about 0.9 million per year. If the annual incidence of 250 million cases from 1950 to 1960 had been maintained there would have been about 25 million malaria deaths attributable to malaria instead of about 15 million that probably occurred during the following decade. A reduction of deaths by 10 million that could be attributed to the control and eradication of malaria took place during the period when the world population increased by 500 million.

The present trends of demographic pressure are only marginally related to activities in the eradication of malaria and represent a worldwide phenomenon that is still not fully understood.

In any case the acceptance of high rate of sickness and mortality in developing countries is unthinkable and the problem of the outrunning of the world's resources in the growth of the population is one that must be solved by the pooling of human intelligence and not by the neglect of human health.[17, 18] During the past quarter of this century the life expectancy in emerging countries has nearly doubled, and the pressure of population has retarded the social and economic advance of tropical areas. A growth of population that occurs after a breakthrough into greater efficiency and productivity acts as a spur for the national economy by creating the expanding cycle of supply and demand. But the situation is different when the population expands faster than the productivity and increases consumption at the expense of saving.

There is little doubt that at least in some countries the problem of the pressure of population on the available resources calls for an urgent and effective policy of family planning. The implementation of such a policy in developing countries depends, like any mass campaign against communicable disease, on the availability of a network of basic health services in addition to mobile units. It seems that the countries that have succeeded best in this field are those where the dynamic and the static approaches have been combined.

The necessary growth of national income and the accumulation of capital for economic development are affected not only by the rapid growth of population; they are frustrated further by the imbalance of international trade that is disadvantageous to underdeveloped areas.

During the past few years Director General Marcolino Candau of WHO has made repeated statements to the annual sessions of the Economic and Social Council of the United Nations in which he has quoted data from the *Third Report on the World Health Situation*.[19] While admitting the great advances achieved in public health practice, Dr. Candau has pointed out that the gap between the rich and the poor countries continues to widen.

Today the rich countries of the world, inhabited by about one third of the human race, have an income per head 10 to 20 times greater than that of the poor countries, which contain two thirds of the world's population.

Apart from a retardation in the progress of eradicating malaria we witness the return of plague and yellow fever, the menace of cholera, the increasing incidence of trypanosomiasis and filariasis, the extension of bilharziasis related to irrigation of new areas, the renewed threat of syphilis and gonorrhea, and the prevalence of malnutrition in many parts of the world.[19]

These reverses are due to the scarcity of medical and health personnel, to administrative shortcomings, to technical difficulties, to the inadequacy of financial resources, and to other factors, not excluding the deterioration of the political situation—the result of overstimulated expectations and of the rising tide of destructive nationalisms.

In the face of today's demographic pressures and their economic consequences there is only one choice left to the underdeveloped world and to the rich countries. The underdeveloped countries must brace themselves for a planned, coordinated, and decisive action aimed at a rapid advance of agricultural and industrial techniques, coupled with education, with rejection of wasteful and antisocial customs, with the improvement of the status of women, with the acceptance of modern methods of population control, and with the utmost austerity. The wealthier countries must realize the dangers of the present unbalanced situation and willingly accept the obligation to provide vastly increased assistance in the form of advisory, technical, and financial help to create sources of knowledge and wealth in the present desert of poverty and ignorance.

No doubt much help has been given to the underdeveloped countries over the past decade, and its value has been tremendous; nevertheless, it is disquieting that this assistance is declining. The reports of the World Bank indicate that in relation to the national income of advanced countries their aid to the underdeveloped part of the world decreased from 0.8% in 1961 to 0.6% to 0.7% during recent years.

There can be little doubt that more aid for developing countries is a moral obligation and a sound policy. Such aid will be of lasting value when the receiving countries realize that it is not a substitute for a national effort. And it is good to know that this concept of "national effort *assisted* by foreign aid" has powerful support among African leaders themselves and is endorsed by the voice of the WHO regional director for Africa.[20]

The first decade of development loudly heralded in 1960 by the United Nations is drawing to a close with an air of disenchantment. Although the dilemma of development has been to a large extent "a study in frustration" there are some signs of improvement. National planning for health within the context of economic and social planning has become an established practice in many developing countries. More attention is being paid to the increase and training of medical manpower, and recent advances in agricultural techniques such as the introduction of new high-yield strains of rice and wheat are spectacular achievements of the Rockefeller and Ford foundations. Thus the expenditure of about 2 million dollars may change the future of millions of people in Asia, America, and Africa! There are attempts at giving a fairer share of international trade to the emerging countries to provide scientific aids to productivity, to promote public investment, and to obtain sounder administrative practices.

This then is the background against which the eradication of malaria from the globe must be judged. We are attempting to wipe out one of the most prevalent diseases over huge tropical areas that have a predominantly rural population still at a low economic and educational level.

To control successfully, if not to eradicate, a disease responsible for so much sickness demands rational planning of health services. This in turn depends on the availability of human and material resources that cannot be deployed without outside assistance.

Financial aid alone, however massive, is only a palliative measure since its success depends on the community's capacity for adaptation to new patterns and trends of events.

15

We have reached a point of no return, and we must persist in our efforts to eliminate the major endemic diseases, even if our strategy must be changed. We cannot afford to lose all that has been gained over the past decade. The new approach may dispel some illusions, but it should not affect our conviction that on the assistance given now to the sick and needy part of mankind depends the future of the human race.

## REFERENCES

1. National Academy of Sciences. *Tropical Health: A Report on a Study of Needs and Resources,* publ. 996. Washington, D.C., National Academy of Sciences, National Research Council, 1962.

2. WHO Report on the Progress of Malaria Eradication Programme, A21/P. & B./1, cyclostyled document. Geneva, WHO, 1968.

3. WHO. *Expert Committee on Malaria: Eighth Report.* Techn. Rep. 205. Geneva, WHO, 1961.

4. WHO. *Expert Committee on Malaria: Ninth Report.* Techn. Rep. 243. Geneva, WHO, 1962.

5. WHO. *Expert Committee on Malaria: Tenth Report.* Techn. Rep. 272. Geneva, WHO, 1964.

6. WHO. *Expert Committee on Malaria: Twelfth Report.* Techn. Rep. 324. Geneva, WHO, 1964.

7. WHO. *Expert Committee on Malaria: Thirteenth Report.* Techn. Rep. 357. Geneva, WHO, 1967.

8. WHO. *Expert Committee on Malaria: Fourteenth Report.* Techn. Rep. 382. Geneva, WHO, 1968.

9. Gonzalez, C. L. *Mass Campaigns and General Health Services.* WHO Public Health Paper 29. Geneva, WHO, 1965.

10. Maegraith, B. G. Unde venis? *Lancet 1:*401, 1963.

11. Maegraith, B. G. Exotic Disease in Practice. London, Heinemann, 1965.

12. Dorolle, P. N. Old plagues in the jet age. *Brit. Med. J. 2:*789, 1968.

13. Bruce-Chwatt, L. J. Malaria research for malaria eradication. *Trans. Roy. Soc. Trop. Med. Hyg. 59:*105, 1965.

14. Sadun, E. H., ed. Research in malaria. *Milit. Med.* (Suppl.) *131,* 1966.

15. Pampana, E. J. *A Textbook of Malaria Eradication.* London, Oxford Univ. Press, 1963.

16. MacKenzie, D. J. M. Personal communication.

17. Russell, P. F. *Man's Mastery of Malaria.* London, Oxford Univ. Press, 1955.

18. Russell, P. F., West, L. S., Manwell, B. D. and MacDonald, G. *Practical Malariology.* London, Oxford Univ. Press, 1963.

19. WHO. *Third Report on the World Health Situation.* Off. Rec. 155. Geneva, WHO, 1967.

20. Quenum, A. Africa at the crossroads. *World Health:* 2-5, 1968.

# DISCUSSION OF PAPER
## BY LEONARD J. BRUCE-CHWATT:
## MALARIA ERADICATION AT
## THE CROSSROADS*

PAUL F. RUSSELL

Staff Member Emeritus
The Rockefeller Foundation
New York, N.Y.

IN 1955 the Eighth World Assembly of WHO decided "that the WHO should take the initiative, provide technical advice, and encourage research and coordination of resources in the implementation of a program having as its ultimate objective the world-wide eradication of malaria." By the end of 1967 this program had resulted directly or indirectly in the eradication of malaria from areas that have a population of about 654 millions. Programs for eradicating malaria were progressing actively in areas with a total population of about 632 millions, and preparatory activities had been started in areas with a total population of about 42 millions. About 364 millions, or only 21%, lived in malarious areas not yet included in the program for the eradication of malaria. (No data are available for mainland China, North Korea, and North Vietnam.)

Remarkable successes have been attained, for example, throughout Europe, in most of North America, much of the Near East, in Formosa, Mauritius, and most of Venezuela. In some countries, as in India, the incidence and death rates from malaria have been dramatically reduced although the eradication of malaria has not yet been accomplished. Viewed in what seems to me logical perspective, the worldwide program for the eradication of malaria of WHO has made notable progress in its first 12 years.

But because about 364 millions live in malarious areas, including most of tropical Africa, which is not yet in the program and where the going will be difficult, and because troublesome problems are being encountered elsewhere in these programs, especially in tropical areas,

*Presented as part of a *Symposium on Malaria* sponsored by The Tropical Disease Center, St. Clare's Hospital, New York, N.Y., and The Merck Company Foundation, Rahway, N.J., held at the Center, May 17, 1969.
This paper was read, in Dr. Russell's absence, by Dr. Norman Stoll.

with a noticeable slowing down of the global program, it seemed advisable to the 20th World Health Assembly in 1967 to request the director general of WHO "to study how best to carry out a re-examination of the global strategy of malaria eradication and to report to the Twenty-first World Health Assembly." Recent epidemics of malaria in Ceylon and in Paraguay have pointed up this need for a careful reexamination of the eradication program.

Director General Marcolino Candau presented a report on this subject to the 21st World Health Assembly in 1968, and his report has had careful study by WHO consultants and staff during the past year. No doubt the subject will be on the agenda of the 22nd World Health Assembly meeting in Boston in the summer of 1969. Reports by Dr. Candau and others suggest that the chief problems confronting the worldwide program for the eradication of malaria today fall into three categories:

1) *Technical.* This means resistance to certain insecticides and drugs by certain strains of species of *Anopheles* and *Plasmodium,* respectively; evasion of insecticides by certain anopheline vectors because of their feeding or resting habits; evasion of protection by certain human populations because of their sleeping or migrating habits; large-scale importation of Plasmodia by human carriers from areas without effective eradication programs.

2) *Socioeconomic.* By this is meant difficulty in obtaining sufficient local and international funds for the eradication of malaria in certain highly malarious countries; difficulty in justifying programs for the eradication of malaria to lay officials because of the paucity of reliable data regarding the impact of malaria and the contrasting impact of its eradication on social and economic conditions and growth in undeveloped malarious countries.

3). *Human fraility.* This category includes programs for the eradication of malaria started hastily without adequate preparations or firm governmental guarantees; lack of trained personnel and training facilities; failure of local organizations to follow WHO guide lines in such a program; failure to maintain effective discipline in spraying and survey operations; inability to overcome the tedium of operations in later stages of a program; failure to push a program through to the eradication of malaria when malaria incidence has fallen to a low level and other diseases therefore seem more important.

18

The problems are numerous and difficult but in most cases not unexpected. Most observers agree that the technical problems will be solved without undue delay. A great deal of malaria research is in progress. The other problems may take years to overcome. But the WHO plan did not envisage the worldwide eradication of malaria within a specified period of time. However the strategy of eradicating malaria did insist that, once started, such a program should be completed as rapidly as possible.

In my opinion the WHO objective of worldwide eradication of malaria is logical and attainable. Obviously one should not set a time limit. There are highly malarious countries where such a program should not yet be started because there are no suitable health organizations, staffs, or guarantees of funds for eradication programs. In such countries WHO can help to develop basic health services and to lay foundations which one day will support programs for the eradication of malaria.

Naturally it will take many years to accomplish the worldwide eradication of malaria but there is no logical reason why the eradication of malaria should not be a continuing effort of WHO, which is not a temporary or a makeshift agency. Let us hope that its several programs of eradication, including that for malaria, will one day achieve worldwide success. Already the world's malarial burden has had an astounding four-fifths reduction, with estimated yearly morbidity totals down from 250 to 50 million, and the annual malaria death rate down from an estimated 2.5 million to less than a million (WHO estimates). I agree with Professor Leonard J. Bruce-Chwatt that "we must persist in our efforts to eliminate the major endemic diseases, even if our strategy must be changed. We can not afford to lose all that has been gained over the past decade."

# RECENT TRENDS IN MALARIA IN THE UNITED STATES*

## GEORGE U. FISHER

Malaria Surveillance Officer
National Communicable Disease Center
Atlanta, Ga.

## INTRODUCTION

ENDEMIC transmission of malaria occurred in what is now the United States from at least the 17th century[1] until 1957, when the last presumed indigenous cases were reported.[2, 3] The public health impact of the disease was impressive, particularly in the southeastern states,[1] where, as late as the early 1930's, parasite rates of 20 to 30% were not uncommon.[4] The rapid decline and eventual disappearance of endemic malaria occurred in the 1940's and early 1950's, as a result of a number of socioeconomic advances and specific measures for the control and eradication of malaria.[1, 5] Imported cases and occasional outbreaks of introduced† malaria continued to occur, but in the late 1950's and early 1960's the number of reported cases rarely exceeded 150 a year.[3] However, since 1966 there has been a marked increase in the number of imported cases in the United States due to the return of infected servicemen from Vietnam.

This paper reviews the recent epidemiologic features of malaria in the United States, including the fatal cases, introduced outbreaks, and infections induced by transfusion.

## GENERAL EPIDEMIOLOGY

The numbers of malaria cases‡ reported in the United States from 1959 through 1965 ranged from 50 to 171 per year, but rose to 764 in 1966, 2,855 in 1967, and 2,610 in 1968; the marked rise was due to an

---

*Presented as part of a *Symposium on Malaria* sponsored by The Tropical Disease Center, St. Clare's Hospital, New York, N. Y. and The Merck Company Foundation, Rahway, N. J., held at the Center, May 17, 1969.

†Introduced malaria: malaria acquired by mosquito transmission from an imported case.

‡A "case" is defined as an individual's first attack of malaria in the United States, whether or not he had experienced previous attacks while outside the country. A subsequent attack in the same individual caused by a different Plasmodium species is counted as an additional case, but repeated attacks caused by the same species are counted as relapses, not additional cases.

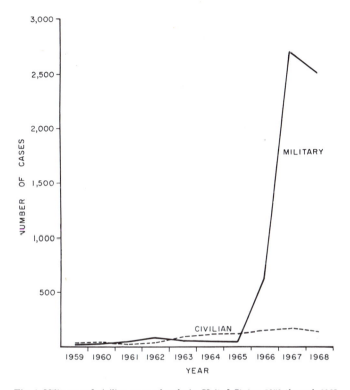

Fig. 1. Military and civilian cases of malaria, United States, 1959 through 1968.

increase in military cases. Civilian infections increased gradually from 38 in 1959 to 157 in 1967, and fell to 123 in 1968 (Figure 1).

Of the 6,229 cases reported in the three-year period of 1966 to 1968, 78.2% were due to *Plasmodium vivax*, 15.4% to *P. falciparum*, 1.1% to *P. malariae*, 0.7% to *P. ovale*, and 1.6% to mixed infections; in 3.0% the *Plasmodium* species was not determined (Table I).

The geographic distribution of the cases reported from 1966 through 1968 is distinctively nonhomogeneous, since most persons who have returned from Vietnam are concentrated on military bases in California, Colorado, Georgia, Kentucky, North Carolina, and Texas These six states accounted for 52% of cases reported during this period. How-

21

TABLE I. MALARIA CASES, UNITED STATES, 1966 THROUGH 1968
BY *PLASMODIUM* SPECIES

| Species | Number | Per cent |
|---------|--------|----------|
| P. vivax | 4,874 | 78.2 |
| P. falciparum | 960 | 15.4 |
| P. malariae | 66 | 1.1 |
| P. ovale | 46 | 0.7 |
| Mixed | 99 | 1.6 |
| Unknown | 184 | 3.0 |
| Total | 6,229 | 100.0 |

TABLE II. INTERVAL FROM RETURN TO UNITED STATES UNTIL ONSET
OF ILLNESS, VIVAX AND FALCIPARUM MALARIA; 1966 THROUGH 1968

| Interval in months | P. vivax Number | Per cent | P. falciparum Number | Per cent |
|--------------------|-----------------|----------|----------------------|----------|
| < 1 | 840 | 18.3 | 556 | 65.0 |
| < 6 | 4,153 | 90.2 | 836 | 97.8 |
| <12 | 4,545 | 98.8 | 850 | 99.4 |
| ≥12 | 57 | 1.2 | 5 | 0.6 |
| Total cases with known interval | 4,602 | | 855 | |

ever, at least one case was reported from every state.

The interval from return to the United States until onset of malaria is known for 4,602 of the 4,874 vivax cases; it was less than 30 days in 18.3%, less than six months in 90.2%, and less than one year in 98.8%. The longest interval was 36 months. In contrast 65.0% of falciparum cases occurred within one month, 97.8% within six months, and 99.4% within 12 months; the longest interval was 21 months (Table II). Civilian physicians are quite likely to encounter the cases which occur during the first month after return from Vietnam, since most servicemen are at home on leave during this period. In addition, cases occurring in veterans are frequently seen by civilian practitioners. From 1966 through 1968, 8.6% of the 6,229 cases were treated in civilian hospitals,

22

TABLE III. MALARIA ATTACK RATES IN THE U.S.A. AMONG ARMY
RETURNEES FROM VIETNAM, BY *PLASMODIUM* SPECIES
AND YEAR OF RETURN, 1966 THROUGH 1968

| Year of return | Cases/100 returnees | | |
|---|---|---|---|
| | All species | P. vivax | P. falciparum |
| 1966 | 1.35 | 1.04 | 0.24 |
| 1967 | 0.94. | 0.80 | 0.11 |
| 1968* | 0.55 | 0.45 | 0.07 |

*1968 rates are preliminary and will increase somewhat as cases among 1968 returnees continue to occur.

14.5% in Veterans Administration hospitals, 74.4% in military hospitals, 1.5 in Public Health Service installations, and 1.0% elsewhere.

Men who had returned to the United States after military service in Vietnam accounted for 5,670 (91%) of the 6,229 cases reported from 1966 through 1968, and it was found then that of these, army men accounted for 5,057 (81.2%). Army troops are currently instructed to take a combination "CP" tablet containing 300 mg. chloroquine base and 45 mg. primaquine base once a week throughout their service in Vietnam and for eight weeks after departure; in addition, most troops are instructed to take 25 mg. diamondiphenylsulfone (DDS) daily in Vietnam and for 28 days after departure. In experimental studies, the effectiveness of the terminal eight week CP regimen in the radical cure of tropical strain *P. vivax* infections has been well demonstrated,[6] but its acceptance in the field by returning troops has been less than optimal.[7]

Among army men returned from Vietnam the malaria attack rate, calculated by year of return to the United States, has declined steadily and significantly since 1966; the same relation holds true if the attack rates are calculated for vivax or falciparum infections alone (Table III). The 1968 attack rates are preliminary and will increase somewhat as cases continue to occur, but they certainly will not exceed the figures for 1967. From data obtained in Vietnam and Fort Bragg, N. C. it is clear that the attack rate varies considerably; it depends on the soldier's unit and rank, as the rates are highest for low-ranking combat troops, particularly small-arms infantrymen, and lowest for officers in support units. The factors responsible for the downward trend in attack rates

TABLE IV. RELAPSE RATES* FOR VIVAX AND FALCIPARUM MALARIA
AMONG ARMY RETURNEES FROM VIETNAM, 1966 THROUGH 1968†

| Year | P. vivax | P. falciparum |
|------|----------|---------------|
| 1966 | 30.9 | 8.2 |
| 1967 | 19.4 | 6.2 |
| 1968† | 5.4 | 1.2 |

*Relapse rate: percentage of cases occurring in a given calendar year that are followed by a second attack caused by the same *Plasmodium* species.
†Rates for 1968 are preliminary and will increase as relapses of 1968 cases continue to occur.

are unknown, but they probably include more complete use of terminal chemoprophylaxis by returning troops and changes in the degree of exposure or use of suppressive therapy in Vietnam.

Civilian malaria has not increased nearly so dramatically as military malaria, but the gradual rise seen in the past 10 years may continue because of the ever expanding role of international travel. The occupation of the affected civilian is varied. In 1968, college students or teachers accounted for 40 civilian cases and merchant seamen for 14; many of the individuals in these two categories were foreign visitors from malarious areas. Foreign nationals accounted for a total of 42 civilian cases, Former Peace Corps volunteers accounted for only six cases in 1968, as opposed to 25 in 1967 and 44 in 1966; almost all of these individuals had served in West Africa. Temporary discontinuation of terminal primaquine treatment for returning West African Peace Corps volunteers from mid-1965 until mid-1967 probably accounted for the bulk of the cases during those years.

From 1966 through 1968, 792 malaria relapses were reported; 644 of these were second attacks, 119 were third attacks, 24 were fourth attacks, 4 were fifth attacks, and one was a sixth attack. Thus a total of 7,021 malaria attacks (6,229 cases, or primary attacks, and 792 relapses) were reported during the three-year period.

Among army personnel returned from Vietnam the relapse rate for vivax cases treated in the United States was much higher in 1966 than in 1967. The 1968 figure, which is preliminary and will rise somewhat as relapses continue to occur, is far below the level for 1967 (Table IV). The substitution in October 1967 of supervised treatment with 15 mg. primaquine base daily for 14 days in place of unsupervised treatment with 1 CP tablet per week for 8 weeks in the radical cure of vivax cases treated in military hospitals in the United States undoubtedly played a role in this decline. The recrudescence rates of falciparum infections have never been appreciable, but the 1967 figure was lower than that for 1966; on the basis of the preliminary data for 1968, it appears that this decline will continue.

## FATALITIES

There were four fatalities from malaria in the United States in 1966, two in 1967, and six in 1968. All were falciparum infections. The falciparum case fatality ratio for the entire three-year period is 1.25%, and by year is 1.63% for 1966, 0.54% for 1967, and 1.74% for 1968. Six of the 12 deaths occurred in persons who had returned from Vietnam, two were merchant seamen, one was the recipient in a transfusion-induced case, one was an American missionary who had returned from Africa, one was an American who had taught in an African college, and one was an American pilot who had flown for a small airline in West Africa.

Detailed case histories were obtained for 11 of the 12 fatalities. All 11 patients had heavy parasitemia (more than 10% of red cells parasitized), and all developed one or more significant complications of their infections (severe hemolysis, cerebral involvement, renal failure, and pulmonary edema). Two of the 11 died without seeking medical care; the remaining nine were hospitalized. The interval from hospitalization to diagnosis was three or more days in four of the nine cases and more than 24 hours in six of the nine. In each of those six cases, falciparum parasites were present on the admission blood smear but were overlooked by the physician or laboratory technician.

Treatment seemed to have little effect on the clinical course of the 11 cases as evidenced by the fact that the average interval from onset of illness to death was 8.3 days for the six patients who received no therapy or who died with less than 24 hours' treatment; the interval was essentially the same, 9.4 days, for the five patients who received treatment for two or more days (average duration of therapy was actually 3.8 days). For the nine patients who received any treatment, the average interval from onset of illness to institution of therapy was 7.1 days (range 2 to 11 days). Several of the patients died of complications of their illness despite clearance of or marked reduction in the level of their parasitemia.

Our experience with falciparum fatalities is thus in keeping with

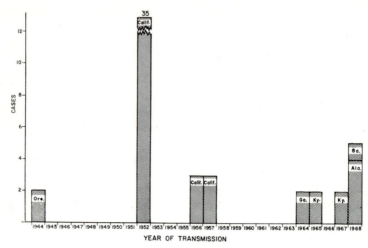

Fig. 2. Malaria introductions, United States, 1944 through 1968. All cases due to *P. vivax*.

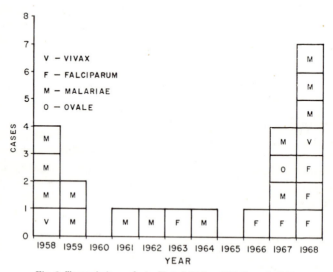

Fig. 3. Transmission malaria, United States, 1958 through 1968.

previous reports[8] that the fatality ratio for falciparum cases is high and may not be appreciably altered by treatment when the duration of untreated illness is long or when the level of parasitemia is very high. Several of our cases, especially those complicated by pulmonary edema, suggest that irreversible tissue damage may occur with severe falciparum malaria and may lead to a fatal complication despite subsequent clearance of parasitemia.

Of all the occupational groups represented in the malaria cases reported in recent years, merchant seamen had the highest fatality ratio for malarial cases: 3.3% from 1966 through 1968 and 4.1% from 1963 through 1968. This distinction stems from two facts: 1) seamen frequently become ill at sea, where appropriate treatment is not readily available, and 2) 51% of the infections in seamen are cause by *P. falciparum*.

## INTRODUCED MALARIA

Mosquito transmission of malaria is possible in the United States since anopheline vectors, imported cases, and a susceptible population are all widespread. Nine well investigated outbreaks of introduced malaria have been reported in the literature since 1944,[2, 3, 9-13] comprising 54 cases, all due to *P. vivax* (Figure 2).* All five of the outbreaks reported since 1964 occurred in the Southeast; four of these occurred on military bases. The number of introduced episodes reported from 1966 through 1968 does not parallel the marked rise in the number of imported cases. This observation, coupled with the over-all rarity and self-limited nature of introduced malaria outbreaks, strongly suggests that epidemiologic and ecologic factors are not favorable for reestablishment of endemicity or even for the occurrence of sizable focal transmission. Among the important deterrent factors are a sensitive surveillance system, prompt detection and treatment of cases (particularly on military bases), and the general high standard of living, which decreases opportunities for contact between mosquito and man.

## TRANSFUSION-INDUCED MALARIA

The number of transfusion-induced malaria cases reported in the United States has increased sharply in recent years, and the species distribution has changed considerably (Figure 3). Of the 21 transfusion-

---

*A few presumptive introduced cases were described in the early 1950's,[14, 15] and additional outbreaks have undoubtedly been unrecognized.

induced cases reported from 1958 through 1968, 12 occurred in the last three years; only one of the first nine cases was caused by P. falciparum, but five of the last 12 were caused by this species. Of the 21 infections, 12 were due to P. malariae, 6 to P. falciparum, 2 to P. vivax, and 1 to P. ovale.

The responsible donor was identified in 11 of the 21 cases, including 10 of the last 12. Five of these were due to P. falciparum, four to P. malariae, and one each to P. vivax and P. ovale. Seven of the donors, including all the P. malariae donors, were immigrants or visitors from endemic areas, usually West Africa. The remaining four donors were American servicemen who had served in Vietnam.

Serologic screening of all donors who had traveled or resided in malarious areas, with the use of indirect fluorescent antibody (IFA) technique, identified the infective donor in all nine cases in which it was applied. Another donor was implicated on epidemiologic grounds alone, and the remaining donor, identified before IFA testing was available, had a positive blood smear.

Attempts were made to demonstrate malaria parasites in nine donors. Two had positive routine blood smears. A third had negative blood smears on several occasions, but his smears finally became positive after he was phlebotomized. A fourth donor had consistently negative peripheral smears, but an aspirate of his bone marrow was positive. A fifth donor had negative blood smears, but his parasitemia was verified by subinoculation of his blood into a human volunteer. Parasites were not demonstrated in the remaining four donors.

The interval between the donor's arrival in the U.S.A. and his donation of the infected blood is known for all 11 cases; it was two or more years for the four P. malariae infections, 36 months for one falciparum infection, 13 months for another falciparum case, and less than one year for the remaining five infections.

Two American men who had served one year in Vietnam and who were the donors responsible for two cases of transfusion-induced falciparum malaria are especially noteworthy, since their infections were asymptomatic for minimum periods of six and 13 months before blood donation, despite the fact that both denied a history of clinical malaria or significant febrile illnesses and despite the fact that they had discontinued their chemoprophylaxis four and 11 months before donation respectively.

Prevention of malaria by transfusion is best achieved by carefully screening potential donors for a history of malaria or of travel to malarious areas. Serologic screening is too expensive and time consuming, and screening of blood smears has the added disadvantage of insensitivity. The American Association of Blood Banks recommends rejection of potential donors who had traveled in malarious areas during the preceding two years.[16] Strict adherence to this rule would have prevented six of the 11 donor-identified cases. However, one falciparum donor and all four malariae donors would have been accepted.

Prevention of transfusion-induced *P. malariae* infections is particularly difficult, since this species may persist throughout the lifetime of the prospective donor. The fact that immigrants or visitors from malaria endemic areas were the donors in all four of our *P. malariae* cases suggests that permanent rejection of these individuals would decrease the incidence of malaria induced by *P. malariae*. Whether such stringent screening would significantly deplete the current pool of donors is unknown.

## CONCLUSION

Malaria is no longer an exotic disease in the United State. Cases should continue to occur in large numbers until the number of American troops serving in Vietnam is significantly reduced. Physicians, laboratory technicians, and public health workers must be aware of this fact in order to prevent undue fatalities and sizable introduced outbreaks. The apparent increase in transfusion-induced malaria indicates a need for careful screening of prospective blood donors.

*R E F E R E N C E S*

1. Russell, P. F. The United States and malaria: Debits and credits. *Bull. N.Y. Acad. Med. 44*:623-53, 1968.
2. Dunn, F. L. and Brody, J. A. Malaria surveillance in the United States, 1956-1957. *Amer. J. Trop. Med. 8*:447-55, 1959.
3. Malaria Surveillance Unit, National Communicable Disease Center. *1966 Annual Summary.* Atlanta, U.S. Public Health Service, 1967.
4. Williams, L. L., Jr. Civil Works Administration, Emergency Relief Administration. Malaria control program in the South. *Amer. J. Public Health 25*: 11-14, 1935.
5. Andrews, J. A., Quinby, G. E., and Langmuir, A. D. Malaria eradication in the United States. *Amer. J. Public Health 40*:1405-11, 1950.
6. Alving, A. S., Johnson, C. F., Tarlov, A. R., Brewer, G. J., Kellermeyer, R. W. and Caroon, P. E. Mitigation of the hemolytic effect of primaquine and enhancement of its action against exo-erythrocytic forms of the Chesson strain

of *Plasmodium vivax* by intermittent regimens of drug administration. *Bull. WHO 22:*621-31, 1960.

7. Skrzypek, G. and Barrett, O., Jr. The problem of vivax malaria in Vietnam returnees. Part II. Malaria chemoprophylaxis survey. *Milit. Med. 133:* 449-52, 1968.

8. Kitchen, S. F. Falciparum malaria. In: *Malariology,* Boyd, M. F., ed. Philadelphia and London, Saunders, 1949, pp. 995-1016.

9. Osgood, S. C. Malaria in the returning soldier. *J.A.M.A. 128:*512-13, 1945.

10. Brunetti, R., Fritz, R. F. and Hollister, A. C. Jr. An outbreak of malaria in California, 1952-1953. *Amer. J. Trop. Med. 3:*779-88, 1954.

11. Luby, J. P., Schultz, M. G., Nowosiwsky, T. and Kaiser, R. L. Introduced malaria at Fort Benning, Georgia, 1964-1965. *Amer. J. Trop. Med. 16:* 146-53, 1967.

12. National Communicable Disease Center: Malaria Surveillance Unit. *1967 Annual Summary.* Atlanta, U.S. Public Health Service, 1968.

13. National Communicable Disease Center: Malaria Surveillance Unit. *1968 Annual Summary.* Atlanta, U.S. Public Health Service, 1969.

14. Fritz, R. F. and Andrews, J. M. Imported and indigenous malaria in the United States, 1952. *Amer. J. Trop. Med. 2:*445-56, 1953.

15. Russell, P. F. World-wide malaria distribution, prevalence, and control. *Amer. J. Trop. Med. 5:*937-65, 1956.

16. *Technical Methods and Procedures of the American Association of Blood Banks.* Chicago, Twentieth Century, 1966.

# THE SEROLOGY OF MALARIA: RECENT APPLICATIONS*

IRVING G. KAGAN, HENRY MATHEWS, AND ALEXANDER J. SULZER

Parasitology Section
National Communicable Disease Center
Atlanta, Ga.

THE serology of malaria has a long and varied history. Only in the last decade have new serologic techniques, such as the indirect fluorescent antibody and hemagglutination tests, been explored for use in solving problems associated with epidemiology, speciation, and diagnosis. In our laboratory, studies on the serology of malaria have been devoted to the evaluation of the indirect hemagglutination (IHA) test as an epidemiologic tool. We believe that malariometric techniques currently employed for the assessment and eradication of malaria are not adequate and that new methods require evaluation. This is especially true in the undeveloped areas of the world where trained manpower to conduct various aspects of case finding, fever and spleen surveys, and slide examination are lacking. We are also studying the indirect fluorescent antibody technique (IFA) with emphasis on its evaluation as a diagnostic method. I shall discuss some of the accomplishments of this program.

## INDIRECT HEMAGGLUTINATION STUDIES

Desowitz and Stein[1] and Stein and Desowitz[2] described an IHA test utilizing formalin and sheep red cells treated with tannic acid and sensitized with antigens from *Plasmodium cynomolgi* and *P. coatneyi*. This test was later used in a field study of malaria immunity in Australian New Guinea.[3, 4] Bray and El-Nahal[5, 6] reported difficulties with this test system and recommended using fresh sheep red cells treated with tannic acid. Mahoney et al.[7] fractionated antigens from the plasmodia of *P. knowlesi* following disruption of the parasites in a French press.

*Presented as part of a *Symposium on Malaria* sponsored by the Tropical Disease Center, St. Clare's Hospital, New York, N.Y., and The Merck Company Foundation, Rahway, N.J., held at the Center, May 17, 1969.

This study was supported in part by the U.S. State Department, Agency for International Development, Participating Agency Service Agreement (PASA) No. RA (HA) 5-68.

Since the IHA test has proved to be useful in seroepidemiologic studies on toxoplasmosis[8, 9] and other parasitic diseases,[10] we attempted to standardize and evaluate the test for malaria.[11] Antigen is prepared from lysing mature schizonts from splenectomized rhesus monkeys infected with the *Anopheles hackeri* strain of *P. knowlesi.** The infected cells are washed and lysed by adding at least 10 volumes of distilled water. The freed plasmodia were washed by centrifugation and stored at −70° C. Blood from a 3-km. monkey could be processed in four hours to yield 5 to 20 ml. of plasmodial sediment. The plasmodia are disrupted by using a cooled French pressure cell,† operated at 20,000 pounds per square inch. The antigen is quite labile and cannot be stored for long periods. Methods for stabilizing the antigen are currently under study.

The IHA test is carried out with human group O erythrocytes that have been tanned with 1:20,000 tannic acid solution and sensitized with malaria antigen. A microtitration method employing 0.05-ml. dilutions of serum is used for antibody titration.

To facilitate the collection of blood, samples obtained on filter paper by finger stick were compared with sera collected by venipuncture. These studies indicate that a finger-stick filter-paper technique yields comparable results and thus can be used to collect specimens in the field. The filter paper ROPACO 1023.038,‡ which met most of the requirements, was cut in 1 × 3-inch rectangles and imprinted with two circles, each 14 mm. in diameter. For field studies the paper rectangles were returned to the diagnostic laboratory in plastic bags with glassine interleaves and a dessicant.

In the laboratory a 13/32-inch disc was punched from within the filled circle. The disc was immersed in 0.2 ml. of phosphate buffered saline solution (PBSS) and agitated twice during the 30-minute soaking period. The disc was removed with a rod, which was rolled over it to express some of the eluate. Approximately 0.13 ml. of eluate could be obtained in this manner. The amount is approximately a 1:16 dilution of the original serum sample.

To evaluate the test for specificity, sera from 61 residents of St. Lawrence Island, Alaska, 11 chronic tuberculosis patients from Atlanta,

*Laboratory of Parasite Chemotherapy, NIH, Chamblee, Ga.
†American Instrument Company, Inc., Silver Spring, Md.
‡Rochester Paper Company, Rochester, Mich.
Use of trade names is for identification only and does not constitute endorsement by the Public Health Service or by the U. S. Department of Health, Education, and Welfare.

32

TABLE I. TESTS ON THE SERA OF INDIVIDUALS HAVING NO
KNOWN HISTORY OF MALARIA

| Source | Titer | | | | | | |
| --- | --- | --- | --- | --- | --- | --- | --- |
| | 0 | 2 | 4 | 8 | 16 | 32+ | Total |
| Normal Alaskans | 54 | 3 | 4 | | | | 61 |
| Syphilis, primary and secondary | 28 | 2 | 8 | 4 | 1 | | 43 |
| Chronic tuberculosis | 5 | 4 | 2 | | | | 11 |
| Parasitology battery | 105 | 13 | 19 | 19 | 6* | 4* | 166 |

*Includes three cases of schistosomiasis and four cases of filariasis.

TABLE II. TESTS OF THE SERA OF INDIVIDUALS WITH
SLIDE-PROVED MALARIA

| Species | Titer | | | | | | |
| --- | --- | --- | --- | --- | --- | --- | --- |
| | 0 | 2 | 4 | 8 | 16 | 32+ | Total |
| P. vivax Honduras | 1 | 0 | 0 | 0 | 2 | 127 | 130 |
| P. falciparum U.S. | 0 | 1 | 0 | 0 | 1 | 15 | 17 |
| Mixed species U.S. | 2 | 0 | 0 | 3 | 3 | 77 | 85 |
| Mixed species U.S., Vietnam | 5 | 0 | 0 | 1 | 2 | 127 | 135 |

Ga., and 43 syphilis patients from throughout the United States were assumed to be from malaria-free areas. A parasitology diagnostic battery of 166 sera were also tested. The sera contained 12 subgroups of specimens known to be serologically positive for echinococcosis, filariasis, schistosomiasis, trichinosis, or other nonmalarious diseases, or negative for all these diseases. Titers of 1:16 and greater were uncommon (0.9%) in sera assumed to be free of antibody against malaria (Table I). In the parasitology diagnostic battery, sera with titers of 1:16 or greater (6%) may represent true positives because they were collected from individuals living in areas where malaria may be endemic.

To evaluate the test for sensitivity, specimens from patients with proved infections were evaluated. Sera from 17 cases of P. falciparum infection primarily represented citizens of the United States who con-

TABLE III. MALARIA ANTIBODY TITERS OBTAINED WITH MILITARY RECRUIT SERA

| Country | Total | Titers | | | | | | | | | | | | | | | | | |
|---|---|---|---|---|---|---|---|---|---|---|---|---|---|---|---|---|---|---|---|
| | | 0 | 2 | 3 | 4 | 8 | 9 | 16 | 27 | 32 | 64 | 81 | 128 | 243 | 256 | 512 | 1,024 | 2,048 | 4,096 |
| United States | 2,237 | 2,203 | 7 | | 7 | 13 | | 7 | | | | | | | | | | | |
| Brazil | 2,681 | 1,979 | 76 | | 68 | 153 | | 134 | | 129 | 59 | | 34 | | 27 | 12 | 8 | 2 | |
| Colombia | 2,961 | 2,162 | 62 | | 108 | 134 | | 166 | | 146 | 93 | | 46 | 2 | 31 | 8 | 2 | 1 | 2 |
| Argentina | 3,077 | 2,877 | | 58 | | | 100 | | 30 | | | 10 | | | | | | | |

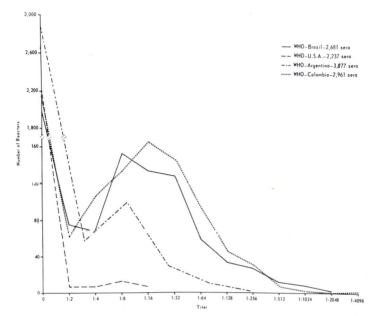

Fig. 1. The frequency distribution of indirect hemagglutination titers for malaria obtained with sera of military recruits.

tracted malaria in a country with known endemic malaria. The sera from 130 persons with *P. vivax* infection were collected in a hyperendemic focus of malaria in Honduras.

Testing sera from persons with malaria diagnosed by blood-smear examination revealed a sensitivity of 96% when a titer of 1:16 or greater was considered a positive reaction (Table II). Sera were collected and stored at —20° C. over a 12-month period without a change of titer.

To evaluate the test for seroepidemiologic studies, 10,956 serum specimens representing four collections of military-recruit sera were tested. The subjects were males varying in age from 18-22 years. The collections consisted of 2,237 sera from the United States, 2,681 from Brazil, 2,961 from Colombia, and 3,077 from Argentina. Table III lists the titers obtained with the military recruit sera. For epidemiologic purposes, a titer of 1:8 or greater was considered positive. This deci-

35

TABLE IV. BRAZIL: COMPARISON OF SEROLOGIC AND BLOOD-SLIDE
RESULTS FOR MALARIA FROM STATES FROM WHICH BOTH DATA
WERE AVAILABLE. STATES ARE RANKED FROM HIGHEST TO
LOWEST VALUE.

| | | Serology | | | Slide examination | |
|---|---|---|---|---|---|---|
| Rank | State code | Name of state | Per cent positive | State code | Name of state | Per cent positive |
| 1 | 3 | Roraima | 100 | 3 | Roraima | 16.8 |
| 2 | 4 | Amazonas | 39.8 | 25 | Goias | 15.7 |
| 3 | 5 | Para | 39.3 | 7 | Maranhão | 15.5 |
| 4 | 2 | Acre | 37.5 | 5 | Para | 14.1 |
| 5 | 12 | Pernambuco | 33.6 | 16 | Bahia | 8.7 |
| 6 | 7 | Maranhão | 27.6 | 8 | Piaui | 6.6 |
| 7 | 25 | Goias | 25.6 | 4 | Amazonas | 5.5 |
| 8 | 24 | Mato Grosso | 25.4 | 2 | Acre | 4.7 |
| 9 | 13 | Alagôas | 25.0 | 18 | Espirito Santo | 4.6 |
| 10 | 8 | Piaui | 23.3 | 24 | Mato Grosso | 3.5 |
| 11 | 17 | Minas Gerais | 18.6 | 17 | Minas Gerais | 3.4 |
| 12 | 16 | Bahia | 17.3 | 22 | Santa Catarina | 3.3 |
| 13 | 10 | Rio Grande do Norte | 15.8 | 9 | Ceará | 2.3 |
| 14 | 22 | Santa Catarina | 12.5 | 21 | Paraná | 2.0 |
| 15 | 11 | Paraiba | 8.8 | 12 | Pernambuco | 1.3 |
| 16 | 19 | Rio de Janeiro | 8.3 | 19 | Rio de Janeiro | 0.6 |
| 17 | 9 | Ceará | 4.6 | 11 | Paraiba | 0.4 |
| 18 | 21 | Paraná | 4.3 | 27 | Guanabara | 0.3 |
| 19 | 15 | Sergipe | 0.0 | 15 | Sergipe | 0.1 |
| 20 | 18 | Espirito Santo | 0.0 | 13 | Alagôas | 0.0 |
| 21 | 27 | Guanabara | 0.0 | 10 | Rio Grande do Norte | 0.0 |

sion was based on the frequency distribution of the titers in each collection as shown in Figure 1. On this basis, the following prevalence of
positive reactors were obtained: United States, 20 (1%) specimens
positive; Brazil, 558 (21%) specimens positive; Colombia, 629 (21%)
specimens positive; and Argentina, 142 (4.6%) specimens positive. The
similar frequency distribution of titers obtained in Brazil and Colombia,
where malaria is widely endemic, and the lower frequency distribution
in Argentina, where malaria endemicity occurs at a low level in limited
parts of the country, suggest that the test is measuring specific malaria
antibody.

The sera positivity rate differs markedly from the rate of malaria
positivity obtained by blood-smear examination in countries where
malaria is endemic. In the United States collection, 99% of the sera
examined were negative. This finding attests to the high specificity of
the test in confirming the absence of malaria in this country. In Brazil
and Colombia the serologic prevalence rate was 21% but the slide pos-

itivity rates for these countries varied from 3 to 5%. The discrepancy in the two methods is probably due to the fact that the IHA test can detect antibody in the blood of an individual many years after infection, whereas the slide method detects only parasites present at the moment the blood is taken for examination. Comparison of serologic and bloodslide results from states in Brazil from which both data were available (Table IV) indicates that 8 of the 10 states with the highest serologic prevalence rates were also among the 10 states with the highest slide-positive rates. The same correlation was found in Colombia. The high correlation suggests that both methods are measuring the prevalence of malaria.

The persistence of the hemagglutination antibody can best be studied in areas where malaria has been eradicated or in individuals who have received radical curative treatment and do not live in endemic areas. A study in an area where malaria has been eradicated was made in Tobago. The last case of autochthonous malaria was reported in Tobago in 1953 and, except for a small introduced outbreak of P. malariae in 1966, the island has remained free of malaria. Through the courtesy of Wilbur Downs 84 sera collected in 1955 in Tobago were titrated for malaria antibody. In 1969 a second collection was made, and 40 of the individuals whose sera were collected in 1955 were bled again. Twenty-three sera were obtained by venipuncture and 13 by the filter-paper method. The prevalence for the 40 individuals fell from 84% to 10% and the geometric mean reciprocal titer from 52.5 to 3.3. Because the minimal detectable titer indicated with filter paper is 1:16, all negative sera are considered 1:2 dilutions for calculating the geometric mean reciprocal titer. The four positive individuals were the oldest people in the sample, and their titers were 1:128, 1:64, 1:16, and 1:16. The prevalence of malaria antibody in the 943 individuals sampled from five areas in Tobago was 1.52% and the geometric mean reciprocal titer was 2:1. These studies indicate that malaria has indeed been eradicated in the island and that antibodies can persist in some individuals for at least 14 years.

A potential use of the serologic method is to delineate the extent of malaria transmission. The question of whether malaria is being transmitted in Nepal above an elevation of 4,000 feet was studied. In a collection of 163 individuals living in villages above this altitude, 22 (13.5%) were positive. Of the 22 positive, 19 were males with a history

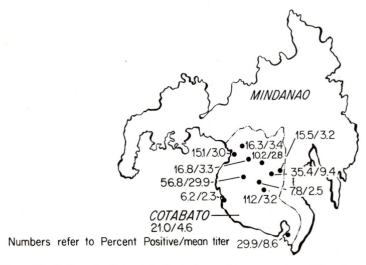

Fig. 2. Distribution of malaria antibodies and geometric mean reciprocal titers for a number of villages in the province of Cotabato on the island of Mindanao, Philippine Republic.

of travel to areas below 4,000 feet. This contrasted with a prevalence of 40% for 502 samples in an endemic area below 4,000 feet. In Ethiopia only 23% of 92 sera collected from individuals living above 6,000 feet were positive compared to 58% of 122 samples collected below 6,000 feet.

The IHA test may also be useful in detecting focal outbreaks of malaria in an endemic area. In a Philippine study done in the province of Cotabato, the prevalence of malarial IHA antibody ranged from 10 to 56%. Two villages with positive serologic rates of 30 and 56% and high geometric mean reciprocal titers were found in a geographical cluster of villages with rates ranging from 10 to 15% and low mean titers (Figure 2). These data suggest that in the two villages with high serologic prevalence, active transmission may be taking place. These malaria "hot spots" can be readily detected with such a survey method.

In Ethiopia serum samples taken in two locations in both wet and dry seasons showed that the positivity rate and the mean titer increased

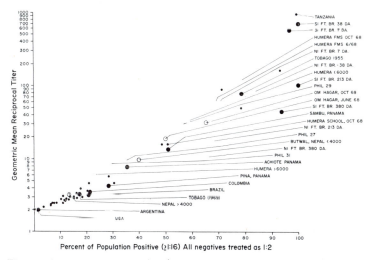

Fig. 3. Relation between the per cent of the population sampled and the geometric mean reciprocal titer for malaria hemagglutination antibody in a number of surveys.

TABLE V. ETHIOPIA: SEASONAL FLUCTUATION OF
MALARIA ANTIBODY LEVELS

| Location | June 1968 (dry) | | October 1968 (wet) | |
|---|---|---|---|---|
| | Per cent positive | Mean titer | Per cent positive | Mean titer |
| Om Hagar School | 50.0 | 18.8 | 65.5 | 30.5 |
| Humera Farms | 68.4 | 56.1 | 78.2 | 113.0 |

markedly in the wet season, the time of peak transmission. This finding indicates the potential use of the IHA test in monitoring seasonal changes in malaria transmission (Table V).

A correlation between the mean geometric reciprocal titer for a survey population and the endemicity of malaria is apparent. To date approximately 20,000 sera, representing collections from the Western Hemisphere, Africa, and Asia have been titrated. These were all "grab samples" and represented many types of populations and epidemiologic situations. The number is large, however, and many of the biases may

39

have been canceled out. This point, however, cannot be assumed and matched populations will be studied. When one plots, on a logarithmic scale, the geometric mean titer versus the per cent positive in the collection, a straight-line relation appears (Figure 3). Serial specimens drawn from a single area but under differing epidemiologic situations move along this line in a predictable manner. This suggests that if a large number of samples are collected from an area, one may readily characterize the endemicity of malaria as hypoendemic, endemic, or holoendemic. Specimens collected at various intervals will make it possible to assess changes in malaria incidence in an area. This assessment can be made rapidly because a collection of several thousand sera can be titrated in a few days by the microtitration method.

In summary: the IHA test may have specialized applications in assessing the prevalence of malaria. Because of the long duration of malaria antibody in a person who has been infected, recent outbreaks of malaria can be detected only by testing young children or by noting a rise in the geometric mean titer over a given period. Since the mean geometric titer and per cent positive of a carefully selected cross section of the population reflects the endemicity of malaria, small surveys in selected areas will readily detect focal outbreaks or a change in the epidemiology of the infection. The technique can be used to delineate the extent of malaria in a country. Other more practical applications, such as monitoring the effect of eradication, or a chemoprophylaxis program in endemic areas, are under study.

## Fluorescent Antibody Studies

The fluorescent antibody (FA) test for malaria was initially introduced by Tobie and Coatney[12] and Voller and Bray.[13] In the last few years a number of workers have made important contributions with this method.[14-24] The FA test is the serologic technique most widely used for the diagnosis of malaria at the present time. Reports by McGregor et al.[25, 26] in Gambia, West Africa, on the use of the fluorescent antibody technique to measure the status of immunity in a population residing in an endemic area have shown that serologic methods may be used to good advantage in the epidemiologic assessment of malaria endemicity.

The FA test, because of technical problems, does not lend itself to mass-screening methods. Nonetheless epidemiologic surveys on relative-

TABLE VI. NUMBER AND PER CENT OF REACTORS TO THREE
PLASMODIUM ANTIGENS AMONG 184 SERA FROM INDIVIDUALS
NOT EXPOSED TO MALARIA AND 49 SERA FROM INDIVIDUALS
WITH A POSITIVE SLIDE DIAGNOSIS*

| Sera group | Titers | Washed-cell thick-smear antigens | | | | | |
|---|---|---|---|---|---|---|---|
| | | P. falciparum No. | % | P. vivax No. | % | P. brasilianum No. | % |
| Donors not exposed | Negative | 157 | 85.3 | 180 | 97.8 | 183 | 99.5 |
| to malaria | 1:4 | 26 | 14.2 | 4 | 2.2 | 1 | 0.5 |
| | 1:16 | 1 | 0.5 | 0 | 0.0 | 0 | 0.0 |
| Donors with positive | Negative | 6 | 12.2 | 4 | 8.2 | 9 | 18.4 |
| slide diag.† | 1:4 | 10 | 20.4 | 4 | 8.2 | 3 | 6.1 |
| | 1:16 | 33 | 67.4 | 41 | 83.6 | 37 | 75.5 |

*Reproduced by permission from: Sulzer, A. J., Wilson, M. and Hall, E. C. Indirect fluorescent antibody tests for parasitic diseases. V. An evaluation of a thick-smear antigen in the IFA test for malaria antibodies. *Amer. J. Trop. Med. 18*:199-205, 1969.

†All sera in this group had previously had titers of at least 1:16 with one of the three antigens. On this second titration, two of these sera had negative reactions with all three antigens.

ly large groups of individuals have been made in Nigeria by Collins et al.[23] and Voller and Bruce-Chwatt.[24]

Use of a soluble antigen fluorescent antibody test with *P. falciparum* and chimpanzee erythrocyte lysates from experimental infections in chimpanzees as antigens adsorbed to cellulose acetate discs may be a more rapid means of performing the fluorescent antibody technique.[27] A stable antigen fractionated by sequential elution with chromatography from a DEAE Sephadex A 25 column gave fractions that were very active in this test. Approximately 50,000 tests can be performed with the amount of antigen normally collected from one infected chimpanzee. This technique is very promising and merits further study because fluorescence is read by a fluorometer, and objective criteria of positive and negative reactions are possible.

We have used a washed-cell thick-smear antigen in all our IFA studies.[28] Washing the parasitized cells removes soluble serum components, especially gamma globulin that may contain malaria antibody and thus may interfere in the test. When such a washed antigen is prepared as a thick smear, the number of plasmodia per field can be controlled. This greatly facilitates the reading of the test results.[29]

The sensitivity and specificity of the test are very high.[29] These parameters were evaluated with a battery of 232 sera, of which 184 were from persons never exposed to malaria and 49 from persons with patent plasmodial infections. All sera were randomized, coded, and

41

TABLE VII. DISTRIBUTION OF TITERS FOR TWO ANTISERA WITH
FOUR ANTIGENS IN THE INDIRECT FLUORESCENT ANTIBODY
(IFA) TEST FOR MALARIA*

| Reciprocal Titer | Plasmodium Antigens | | | | | | | |
|---|---|---|---|---|---|---|---|---|
| | P. vivax | | P. falciparum | | P. brasilianum§ | | P. fieldi | |
| | E.T.† | MOR.‡ | E.T. | MOR. | E.T. | MOR. | E.T. | MOR. |
| Negative | | | | 6 | | 4 | | 2 |
| 4 | | | | 14 | | 9 | 2 | 3 |
| 16 | 16 | 9 | 22 | 27 | | 25 | 10 | 8 |
| 64 | 29 | 30 | 28 | 2 | | | | |
| 256 | | 1 | | | 6 | | | |
| 1,024 | | | | | 34 | | | |
| 4,096 | | | | | 2 | | | |
| Total replicates | 45 | 40 | 50 | 49 | 42 | 38 | 12 | 13 |

*Reproduced by permission from: Sulzer, A. J., Wilson, M. and Hall, E. C. Indirect fluorescent antibody tests for parasitic diseases. An evaluation of a thick-smear antigen in the IFA test for malaria antibodies. *Amer. J. Trop. Med. 18*:199-205, 1969.

†*Plasmodium malariae* demonstrated in circulating blood. Mother of an infant with congenital malaria.

‡District medical officer, Sepik, New Guinea. Reported *Plasmodium vivax* infection with treatment one year prior to sampling.

§*P. brasilianum* antigen was used as an equivalent to *P. malariae*.

tested with antigens prepared from *Plasmodium vivax, P. falciparum,* and *P. brasilianum,* the latter used as a substitute for *P. malariae.* As seen in Table VI only one of the sera from the nonexposed group had a positive reaction at 1:16 with the *P. falciparum* antigen. Specificity is, therefore, greater than 99%. The false positive rates with the *P. brasilianum* and *P. vivax* antigens at the 1:4 dilution were less than 3%, but 14% of the sera reacted with the *P. falciparum* antigen. For this reason a positive reaction at 1:4 with any antigen species is regarded as a questionable positive, and the lowest acceptable diagnostic titer for malaria is 1:16.

The 49 positive sera included in this battery had been tested previously and found to have low antibody concentration. Sera of low titer were chosen so that the most rigorous test of sensitivity might be made. The inclusion of many sera of high antibody titers, which are readily detected by serologic tests, would give a sensitivity rate that might be misleading. As noted in the footnote to Table VI, two of the sera retested gave no reaction at the 1:16 dilution with any of the antigens. This constituted a false negative rate of less than 5%. All other sera were positive at 1:16 with at least one antigen. Some sera reacted only with their homologous antigen. For a diagnostic procedure with the highest sensitivity homologous antigens of the human species should be employed. For this reason we maintain P. *vivax* and P. *falciparum* in Aotus sp. and Ateles sp. monkeys respectively. If homologous human plasmodial antigens are not available, however, a P. *vivax* antigen may be used. With this antigen, the specificity would be better than 95%; the sensitivity with sera of low titer about 92%.

Reproducibility of titers with the thick-smear antigen on a test-to-test basis is excellent (Table VII). Two positive sera were tested with each of four antigen species many times. All titers were replicated within plus or minus one fourfold dilution except for the MOR. serum tested with the P. *falciparum* antigen.

The IFA test can be used to determine the infecting plasmodium species when one cannot make a determination with stained blood slides.[30] Etiologic diagnosis may be difficult because the parasites may have been distorted by the effect of drugs, the parasitemia too scanty to reveal diagnostic forms, or the species identification in doubt because the slides were improperly prepared. The method may be used to detect responsible donors in transfusion malaria.

An evaluation of species identification was made with 206 sera from 93 military personnel who, after returning from Southeast Asia, relapsed with malaria infections. Both acute and convalescent sera were tested. In each case, the infecting plasmodium species was determined by stained blood slides. Since only P. *vivax* and P. *falciparum* infections were involved, antigens of these two species alone were employed in the evaluation.

Comparisons were made on the basis of fourfold titer differences with the two antigens. The species representing the antigen that gave the highest titer was designated as the infecting species. When matched with the slide results, the correct species was identified serologically for 89% of the specimens. Six per cent gave the same titer for both antigens; one case (0.5%) was misdiagnosed, and 5% were negative. Species determinations have become routine in our laboratory and have proved very useful in transfusion malaria and in correcting some misdiagnoses based on improperly stained blood films.

The rise and fall of antibody titer in returning military personnel may be useful diagnostically in that high antibody titer may indicate recent or current infection, especially if there is no history of recent treatment.[31] Sera from 69 individuals reporting to a military hospital in the United States with clinical cases of malaria were studied. In the first two weeks after onset of symptoms the titers were relatively high, with a geometric mean of 1:184. After six months of treatment the titers fell to a mean of 1:9. In this group only one serum had a titer of 1:256. These data clearly suggest that a titer of 1:256 in a returning soldier indicates recent malaria infection. If there is no history of treatment and if parasitemia is not detectable an antibody titer of 1:256 may be regarded as serologic evidence of current malaria infection.

In summary: when a washed-cell thick-smear antigen is used, the IFA test for malaria gives good reproducibility, sensitivity, and specificity. The infecting species of malaria can be identified serologically. When malaria is suspected but definitive diagnosis cannot be made by stained blood film, IFA test results may be useful. For maximum diagnostic sensitivity, homologous plasmodial species antigen should be used. Human plasmodial species from infections in Aotus and Ateles monkeys make excellent antigen. *P. brasilianum* appears to give serological results identical with those of *P. malariae* antigen.

## Summary

Studies in progress on the application of the indirect hemagglutination test for epidemiologic purposes of malaria are outlined. The test is both sensitive and specific, and antibody can be titrated from plasma eluted from filter paper. The technique may be used to determine serologic positive rates in a population, to determine the extent of malaria transmission, and to characterize the endemicity of malaria.

The indirect fluorescent antibody test is also under evaluation for diagnostic purposes. Evaluation of sensitivity and specificity using a washed-cell thick-smear antigen indicates a procedure of high sensitivity and specificity. Species indentification by using homologous malarial antigen is possible. The significance and duration of antibody in individuals who have undergone radical cure by chemotherapy shows a fall in titer to levels below 1:256 in six months. Human plasmodial species in monkeys may be used as antigen.

## Acknowledgments

We extend thanks to all the individuals who have collaborated with us to make these studies possible: to Dr. W. A. Rogers for initiating many of these studies when he was in charge of the Malaria Serology Laboratory; to Dr. Tom Vernon for his collaboration in Nepal; to Dr. Sam Putnam for his collaboration in Ethiopia; to Dr. A. S. Evans, director of the WHO Reference Serum Bank at Yale University for making the Philippine and Western Hemisphere collections available; and to Dr. George Fisher for his help in Tobago.

## REFERENCES

1. Desowitz, R. S. and Stein, B. A tanned red cell hemagglutination test using *Plasmodium berghei* antigen and homologous antisera. *Trans. Roy. Soc. Trop. Med. Hyg. 56*:257, 1962.

2. Stein, B. and Desowitz, R. S. The measurement of antibody in human malaria by a formalized tanned cell haemagglutination test. *Bull. WHO 30*:45-49, 1964.

3. Desowitz, R. S. and Saave, J. J. The application of the haemagglutination test to a study of the immunity to malaria in protected and unprotected population groups in Australian New Guinea. *Bull. WHO 32*:149-59, 1965.

4. Desowitz, R. S., Saave, J. J. and Stein, B. The application of the indirect haemagglutination test in recent studies on the immuno-epidemiology of human malaria and the immune response in experimental malaria. *Milit. Med. 131*: (Suppl.): 1157-66, 1966.

5. Bray, R. S. and El-Nahal, H. M. S. Antibody estimation by passive haemagglutination in malaria and leishmaniasis. *Trans. Roy. Soc. Trop. Med. Hyg. 60*:423-24, 1966.

6. Bray, R. S. and El-Nahal, H. M. S. Indirect haemagglutination test for malaria. *Nature 212*:83, 1966.

7. Mahoney, D. F., Redington, B. C. and Schoenbechler, M. J. The preparation and serologic activity of plasmodial fractions. *Milit. Med. 131*: (Suppl.): 1141-51, 1966.

8. Walls, K. W., Kagan, I. G. and Turner, A. Studies on the prevalence of antibodies to *Toxoplasma gondii*. I. US military recruits. *Amer. J. Epidem. 85*: 87-92, 1967.

9. Walls, K. W. and Kagan, I. G. Studies on the prevalence of antibodies to *Toxoplasma gondii*. 2. Brazil. *Amer. J. Epidem. 86*:305-13, 1967.

10. Cuadrado, R. R. and Kagan, I. G. The prevalence of antibodies to parasitic diseases in sera of young army recruits from the United States and Brazil. *Amer. J. Epidem. 86*:330-40, 1967.

11. Rogers, W. A., Fried, J. A. and Kagan, I. G. A modified, indirect microhemagglutination test for malaria. *Amer. J. Trop Med. 17*:804, 1968.

12. Tobie, J. E. and Coatney, G. R. Fluorescent antibody staining of human malaria parasites. *Exp. Parasit. 11*:128-32, 1961.

13. Voller, A. and Bray, R. S. Fluorescent antibody staining as a measure of malarial antibody. *Proc. Soc. Exp. Biol. Med. 110*:907-10, 1962.

14. Kuvin, S. F., Tobie, J. E., Evans, C. B., Coatney, G. R. and Contacos, P. A. Antibody production in human malaria as determined by the fluorescent antibody technique. *Science 135*:1130-31, 1962.

15. Kuvin, S. F., Tobie, J. E., Evans, C. B., Coatney, G. R. and Contacos, P. A. Fluorescent antibody studies on the course of antibody production and serum gamma globulin levels in normal volunteers infected with human and simian malaria. *Amer. J. Trop. Med. 11*:129-436, 1962.

16. Garnham, P. C. C., Pierce, A. E. and Roitt, I. *Immunity to Protozoa*. Oxford, Blackwell, p. 3, 1963.

17. Tobie, J. E. Detection of malaria antibodies—immunodiagnosis. *Amer. J. Trop. Med. 13* (Suppl.): 195-203, 1964.

18. Corradetti, A., Verolini, F., Sebastiani, A., Proietti, A. M. and Amati, L. Fluorescent antibody testing with

sporozoites of plasmodia. *Bull. WHO 30*:747-50, 1964.

19. Voller, A. Fluorescent antibody methods and their use in malaria research. *Bull. WHO 30*:343-54, 1964.

20. Collins, W. E., Skinner, J. C., Guinn, E. A., Dobrovolny, C. G. and Jones, F. E. Fluorescent antibody reactions against six species of simian malaria in monkeys from India and Malaysia. *J. Parasit. 51*:81-84, 1965.

21. Collins, W. E., Jeffrey, G. M., Guinn, E. and Skinner, J. C. Fluorescent antibody studies in human malaria. IV. Cross reactions between human and simian malaria. *Amer. J. Trop. Med. 15*:11-15, 1966.

22. Lunn, J. S., Chin, W., Contacos, P. A. and Coatney, A. R. Changes in antibody titers and serum protein fractions during the course of prolonged infections with vivax or with falciparum malaria. *Amer. J. Trop. Med. 15*:3-10, 1966.

23. Collins, W. E., Skinner, J. C. and Coifman, R. E. Fluorescent antibody studies in human malaria. V. Response of sera from Nigerians to five *Plasmodium* antigens. *Amer. J. Trop. Med. 16*:568-71, 1967.

24. Voller, A. and Bruce-Chwatt, L. J. Serological malaria surveys in Nigeria. *Bull. WHO 39*:883-97, 1968.

25. McGregor, I. A., Carrington, S. and Cohen, S. Treatment of East African *P. falciparum* malaria with West African human γ-globulin. *Trans. Roy. Soc. Trop. Med. Hyg. 57*:170-75, 1963.

26. McGregor, I. A., Williams, K., Voller, A. and Billewicz, W. Z. Immunofluoresence and the measurement of immune response to hypoendemic malaria. *Trans. Roy. Soc. Trop. Med. Hyg. 59*:395-414, 1965.

27. Sadun, E. H. and Gore, R. W. Mass diagnostic test using *Plasmodium falciparum* and chimpanzee erythrocyte lysate. *Exp. Parasit. 23*:277-85, 1968.

28. Sulzer, A. J. and Wilson, M. The use of thick-smear antigen slides in the malaria indirect fluorescent antibody test. *J. Parasit. 53*:1110-11, 1967.

29. Sulzer, A. J., Wilson, M. and Hall, E. C. Indirect fluorescent antibody tests for parasitic diseases. V. An evaluation of a thick-smear antigen in the IFA test for malaria antibodies. *Amer. J. Trop. Med. 18*:199-205, 1969.

30. Gleason, N. N., Wilson, M., Sulzer, A. J. and Runcik, K. Serological speciation of *Plasmodium vivax* and *P. falciparum* infections by the malaria IFA test. *Amer. J. Trop. Med.* In press.

31. Wilson, M., Sulzer, A. J. and Runcik, K. The relationship of malaria antibody titer to parasitemia as measured by the indirect fluorescent antibody test. *Amer. J. Trop. Med.* In press.

46

# RENAL AND HEMATOLOGIC COMPLICATIONS OF ACUTE FALCIPARUM MALARIA IN VIETNAM *

CRAIG J. CANFIELD

Chief, Clinical Malaria Research Unit
Walter Reed Army Institute of Research
Washington, D.C.

MALARIA is a major medical problem of U.S. Army personnel in Vietnam. Although it ranks after diarrheal and common respiratory disease as a medical cause for admission to a treatment facility,† malaria requires longer hospitalization for treatment and convalescence and is probably the major cause of medical disability of the military population.

During the four-year interval from 1965 through 1968 there were more than 26,000 acute attacks of malaria in U. S. Army personnel in Vietnam (Table I). Naval, marine, and air force personnel are reported separately and thus are not included in these statistics. Most of the attacks were due to *Plasmodium falciparum*. The increase in malaria since 1965 reflects the increase in the number of men assigned to Vietnam and hence exposed to malaria. There have been 53 deaths in army personnel during this 4-year interval directly attributable to malaria and its complications. The major complications associated with a fatal outcome were acute renal insufficiency, cerebral malaria, and pulmonary edema. In individual cases, more than one of these complications were often present concurrently. It was therefore difficult to determine which was predominant. The decreased rate of mortality since 1965 was probably influenced by a change in antimalarial drug therapy. During the fall of 1965 the prevalence of resistance to chloroquine was not recognized and many patients were treated with chloroquine alone until resistance was documented. Then additional drugs were administered. Since 1966, combination therapy has been employed when the diagnosis of falciparum malaria was established—usually with quinine, pyrimethamine, and diaminodiphenylsulphone (DDS).

*Presented as part of a *Symposium on Malaria* sponsored by The Tropical Disease Center, St. Clare's Hospital, New York, N.Y. and The Merck Company Foundation, Rahway, N.J., held at the Center, May 17, 1969.
†Department of the Army, Office of the Surgeon General, Medical Statistics Agency.
This paper is Contribution No. 591 from the Army Research Program in Malaria.

TABLE I—MALARIA CASES IN U.S. ARMY PERSONNEL IN VIETNAM*

|  | Number | Deaths |
|---|---|---|
| 1965 | 1,972 | 16 |
| 1966 | 6,655 | 14 |
| 1967 | 9,124 | 11 |
| 1968 | 8,616 | 12 |
| Total | 26,367 | 53 |

*Medical Statistics Agency, Office of The Surgeon General, U. S. Army Medical Corps.

TABLE II—ACUTE FALCIPARUM MALARIA IN VIETNAM:
MAJOR COMPLICATIONS

| Authors: | Sheehy and Reba[1] | Blount* |
|---|---|---|
| Years | 1965-1966 | 1966-1967 |
| Total Cases | 3,300 | 2,003 |
| Major complications: |  |  |
| Renal | 19 | 8 |
| Cerebral | 16 | 24 |
| Pulmonary | 3 | 0 |
| Hematologic | * | 21 |

*Not listed.

Many other patients developed complications but survived. No comprehensive documentation of complications is available for the U.S. Army. However several Army Medical Corps officers have accumulated data pertinent to the relative occurrence of complications in patients with malaria. Two separate series of patients are shown in Table II.[1, 2] The data from both of these reports were collected at the 85th Evacuation hospital at Qui Nhon during successive years of observation. The major complication recorded during the year 1965-1966 was acute renal insufficiency; 19 patients with this complication were seen. Several of the patients were evacuated to facilities for specialized treatment in the Philippines or Japan. However, during 1966-1967 only eight patients with renal complications were seen and none was evacuated for renal insufficiency. They had only mild azotemia and hemoglobinuria. The decreased incidence of renal insufficiency requiring dialysis has remained at a low level.

No comparable decrease in incidence has been reported for cerebral malaria. Criteria for diagnosis, however, are less rigid for cerebral malaria than for renal failure and it is therefore difficult to evaluate comparative changes in rates.

The other serious complication which has led to a fatal outcome is pulmonary edema. Patients with pulmonary edema have been observed who had no evidence of overhydration or cardiac decompensation.[3] The condition is usually rapidly fatal and only an occasional patient has survived. Hematologic complications do not usually lead to death, but do prolong convalescence; they will be discussed later.

## RENAL INSUFFICIENCY

Blackwater fever is a urinary manifestation of acute malaria. This term, however, refers simply to the passage of hemoglobin in the urine secondary to rapid or severe lysis of erythrocytes. The presence of blackwater fever in a patient with acute falciparum malaria does not imply an abnormality of renal function; rather it means that the plasma haptoglobin level has been exceeded and that free hemoglobin, or the products of its breakdown, are being excreted by the kidney. Blackwater fever is not necessarily associated with elevation of the blood urea nitrogen.

Oliguric renal failure is a functional abnormality—the decreased production of urine. Decreased production of urine does not necessarily accompany overt uremia in malaria; therefore we prefer the more simple term of acute renal insufficiency to describe the major renal complication of malaria.

Several features have been regularly observed in patients with acute renal insufficiency associated with falciparum malaria.[1, 4, 5, 6]

Of these, intense parasitemia and severe hemolysis with hemoglobinuria are observed most frequently. In one series of 18 patients, nine had more than 10% of their red cells parasitized and 14 had severe hemolysis and hemoglobinuria.[6] In these patients and others hemoglobinuria was present prior to the administration of quinine, and patients were subsequently treated with quinine without apparent increase in hemolysis.[4-8]

Dehydration is also commonly reported. Uncertainty of fluid-elec-

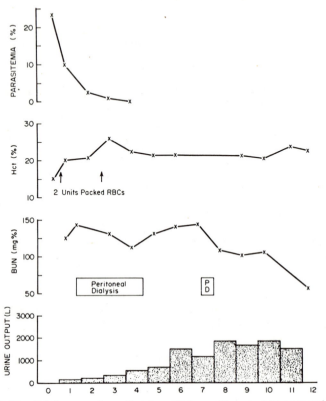

Fig. 1. The clinical course of a patient from Vietnam with acute falciparum malaria and renal insufficiency.

trolyte status makes this feature much more difficult to assess. Preinfection body weight is usually not known, urinary specific gravity is not increased as in simple dehydration, and hyponatremia or relative water excess is common even in uncomplicated malaria infections.[9]

The fourth feature, hypotension, is usually not recorded after the patient is hospitalized and placed in the supine position. However, orthostatic hypotension is common and may contribute to the pathogenesis of renal insufficiency.[10]

Finally, coagulation defects have been found in patients with recrudescent falciparum malaria in the United States.[11] The degree of abnormality was usually related to the severity of the illness. In Vietnam, five patients with renal insufficiency due to malaria have been tested. for consumptive coagulopathy and four had evidence of this process.[6]

The relation between these five features and the pathogenesis of acute renal insufficiency is unknown. Some of these features are known to be regularly present or essential for the production of acute renal failure in experimental animals. For example, in the methemoglobin ferrocyanide[12] and glycerol models[13] of experimental acute renal failure, heme pigments in plasma and urine, dehydration, and sodium depletion are necessary for the regular production of renal failure. The relation between the numerous tubular casts in the experimental models and in patients with renal insufficiency secondary to malaria has not been defined.

Microscopic examination of percutaneous biopsy specimens from patients recovering from renal insufficiency associated with malaria showed minimal histologic alterations: hyaline and hemoglobin casts, tubular atrophy, and focal fibrosis.[10] Iron-positive pigment was present in the epithelium of tubules and in interstitial cells.

Renal function studies have been performed in patients with varying degrees of functional impairment and azotemia. In nonazotemic patients (Thai civilian[9] and American military[14]) renal function usually has been normal. Creatinine or urea clearances and PAH clearances were usually normal with normal filtration fractions.

Figure 1 illustrates some of the characteristics of the disease; it shows the clinical course of a 21-year-old patient who had acute falciparum malaria and renal failure. After a five-day illness, the patient was admitted to an army hospital in Vietnam. He had intense parasitemia (23 per cent) and severe hemolysis (hematocrit of 15 per cent, gross hemoglobinemia, and hemoglobinuria). He also had hypovolemia and hyponatremia, and his initial supine blood pressure was 92/74 mm. Hg. He had azotemia and oliguria. No tests for consumptive coagulopathy were performed.

The patient was treated with quinine, sulforthodimethoxine (Fanasil), and pyrimethamine. Subsequently he was given peritoneal dialysis for renal insufficiency. During the acute stages of the disease there was only a minimal decrease in the blood urea nitrogen with almost

51

three days of continuous dialysis. A subsequent dialysis during convalescence was followed by a prompt decrease in the blood urea nitrogen.

The initial slow response could have been due to decreased efficiency of dialysis or to an increase in the patient's catabolic rate. A markedly increased catabolic rate is suggested by the increased urinary excretion of urea nitrogen during the acute illness.[10] Special studies in this and other patients have also shown decreased efficiency of dialysis which returns to normal as parasitemia declines.[5, 8]

Quinine given intravenously in reduced amounts is recommended for patients from Vietnam who have malaria and acute renal insufficiency. The presence of hemoglobinuria is not a contraindication. The patient described above received 2.1 gm. of quinine during his first two days in the hospital. Quinine administered intravenously during a 1 hour period produced peak concentrations greater than 15 mg./l. but did not produce significant electrocardiographic changes. We now recommend that patients with falciparum malaria and renal insufficiency be treated with quinine (600 gm. per 24 hours) by constant infusion for several days until parasites have been eradicated and oral medication is tolerated, The patient should also be given pyrimethamine to decrease the possibility of relapse.

In the case that has just been described the renal insufficiency was managed with peritoneal dialysis. This treatment is satisfactory for most patients if used early in the course of the disease. Many other patients in Vietnam have been treated with hemodialysis.[4, 6] Prior to deployment of the 629th Renal Unit to Vietnam in mid 1966, patients with renal insufficiency were taken out of the country. There were four deaths during evacuation or shortly thereafter. Since a renal unit was established in Saigon, earlier treatment has been possible and only one death has occurred during evacuation.

Earlier recognition of impending renal insufficiency in patients with severe infections and hemoglobinuria at the evacuation or field hospital has also been important. Patients so identified are treated with osmotic diuresis,[2] which has altered the progression of renal insufficiency in other conditions.[15]

In summary, acute renal insufficiency in patients from Vietnam who have falciparum malaria is generally associated with severe infections, severe hemolysis, derangements in electrolyte balance, hypotension, and consumptive coagulopathy. Prompt treatment with reduced amounts of quinine given intravenously and osmotic diuresis or dialysis has resulted in improved survival rates.

## HEMATOLOGIC COMPLICATIONS

Hematologic complications of acute falciparum malaria include consumptive coagulopathy, severe or prolonged anemia, and leukopenia.

Coagulation studies, including specific factor assays, were performed on 31 American soldiers who had recurrences of acute falciparum malaria in this country.[11] All patients had abnormal prothrombin times or partial thromboplastin times, and 22 of the 31 had platelet counts of less than 150,000. The factor assays showed that V, VII, VIII, and X were depleted. Fibrinogen concentrations less than 200 mg./100 ml. were found in only 10 patients although the serial thrombin time was abnormal in all but two.

As noted above, the degree of abnormality of these coagulation studies is directly related to the severity of illness in each patient. Subsequent studies in human volunteers infected with falciparum malaria treated when symptoms first developed showed only mild thrombocytopenia.[16] Treatment with heparin of patients seriously ill with malaria who had abnormal coagulation produced clinical improvement and partial correction of the coagulopathy within 12 to 24 hours. Concomitant antimalarial drug therapy confounds the role of anticoagulant therapy. Thrombi in various organs of moribund malaria patients suggest that there is a relation between consumptive coagulopathy and the pathophysiology of the disease. The depletion of coagulation factors may be an indication of thrombosis and correction with heparin should probably be attempted.

Approximately 20% of patients with acute falciparum malaria develop significant anemia, with hematocrit levels of less than 35%. The anemia may persist and may require prolonged convalescence.

The degree of anemia is usually related to the severity of the infection. However, patients may have mild infections and severe anemia; some in this group have erythrocytes deficient in glucose-6-phosphate dehydrogenase. Demonstration of this enzyme deficiency is complicated by the preferential lysis of deficient cells in infection and by hemolysis caused by antimalarial drugs. Thus, during the period of

53

TABLE III.—ACUTE FALCIPARUM MALARIA, FERROKINETIC STUDIES

| Patient | Serum iron ($\mu g./100\ ml.$) | Plasma iron clearance (hr.) | Plasma iron Transport rate ($mg./day/70\ kg.\ man$) |
|---|---|---|---|
| 1 | 98.0 | 1.42 | 39.9 |
| 2 | 90.0 | 1.65 | 29.1 |
| 3 | 35.4 | 0.33 | 69.8 |
| 4 | 38.0 | 0.68 | 31.9 |
| 5 | 37.7 | 0.38 | 47.0 |
| 6 | 30.8 | 0.55 | 26.1 |
| 7 | 35.0 | 0.56 | 42.5 |
| 8 | 57.0 | 0.90 | 42.5 |
| 9 | 72.0 | 0.63 | 70.1 |
| 10 | 25.1 | 0.44 | 29.6 |
| 11 | 41.1 | 0.95 | 30.7 |
| 12 | 30.0 | 0.44 | 41.1 |
| 13 | 19.4 | 0.47 | 22.6 |
| Mean | 46.9 | 0.72 | 40.2 |
| Normal range | 70-160 | 1-2 | 20-42 |

severe anemia and before a new population of cells has been generated, screening tests may not reveal the defect. Also, demonstration of other red cell abnormalities that might be associated with hemolysis, such as deficiency of glutathione reductase, is impractical in Vietnam.

A study of 13 patients with acute falciparum malaria treated with quinine, pyrimethamine and Fanasil showed a mean decrease of 10 per cent in the hematocrit during the first two weeks of illness. A significant reticulocyte response did not occur until the 10th day of treatment.

Ferrokinetic studies were performed in these patients. Serum iron concentrations, plasma iron clearance times, and iron turnover data are shown in Table III. The data were obtained prior to treatment and show a normal ferrokinetic response to a demand for red cell formation. Serum iron concentrations were generally decreased. There was rapid clearance of the labeled iron, and calculated turnover rates were at the upper limit of normal. Subsequent red cell incorporation studies during antimalarial therapy are shown in Figure 2. Seven of the 13 patients had abnormally decreased incorporation of $Fe^{59}$ into red blood

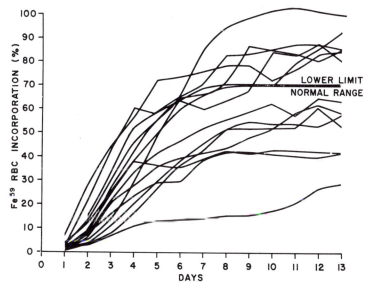

Fig. 2. Red blood cell incorporation of $Fe^{59}$ in 13 patients from Vietnam with acute falciparum malaria during treatment with quinine, pryrimethamine, and sulforthodimethoxine.

cells. This abnormality could be due either to ineffective erythropoeisis or to preferential hemolysis of young cells. Preferential lysis of older cells would have produced a normal initial incorporation with a subsequent decrease. Random hemolysis would not produce the observed degree of abnormality without a marked decrease in hematocrit.

Further studies of anemia were designed to determine if the ferrokinetic abnormality might be due to the antifolic acid actions of pyrimethamine on the maturation of red blood cells.[17] Thirty-six patients were studied with 9 in each of 4 groups. All patients received quinine and DDS. The patients in groups 1 and 2 received pyrimethamine, 50 mg. daily for three days, and those in groups 1 and 3 received 6 mg. of folinic acid every 12 hours intramuscularly for 12 days. The study was double blind, placebos being administered when appropriate. $Fe^{59}$ was given on the fourth day of study.

There was little difference in the average hematocrit decrease or

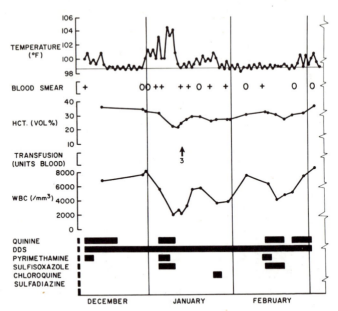

Fig. 3. The prolonged clinical course of a patient from Vietnam who had recurring falciparum malaria despite a variety of therapeutic regimens, finally treated with trimethoprim.

reticulocyte response in the four groups. However, the rate of clearance of parasites was more rapid in the two groups that received pyrimethamine regardless of treatment with folinic acid.

The data obtained from the ferrokinetic studies show that plasma-iron transport rates were generally elevated but there was no significant difference between the treated groups. The plasma-iron transport rates were even greater than in the previous study and inversely proportional to the hematocrit on the day of the study. Although red blood cell incorporation was minimally decreased from normal in one third of the patients, the differences were equally distributed between the various treatment groups. The degree of abnormality was much less than in the previous study and suggested an improvement in the incorporation of iron after the fourth day of treatment.

We interpret the data as follows: during treatment for acute falciparum malaria the patients have an appropriate initial response to hemolysis, quantities of free iron are removed avidly from the plasma.

56

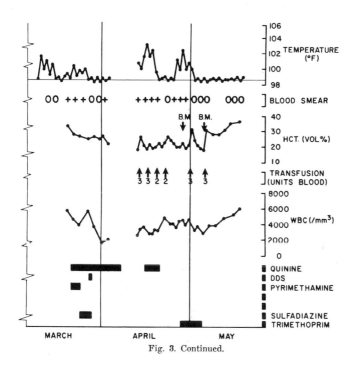

Fig. 3. Continued.

Formation or release of newly formed erythrocytes is impaired until the disease is controlled. In the usual patient who has only mild anemia pyrimethamine probably does not contribute significantly to this delayed erythrokinetic response.

However, pyrimethamine may inhibit erythropoeisis in the patient who has severe hemolysis and in whom the demand for red blood cell production is greatest. Study of the most anemic patient in each of the four different treatment regimens in the study described above showed that the patients who received pyrimethamine had a delay of three to four days in reticulocyte response when compared to the patients who did not receive pyrimethamine. The delay in reticulocytosis was not completely corrected by folinic acid. The erythropoetic response in the patients who received folinic acid was earlier than expected but the early response could have been due to the greater stimulus for

57

the production of red cells from the severe hemolysis.

These observations suggest a dependent relation between the administration of pyrimethamine and a delayed recovery from anemia in those patients who have had moderately severe hemolysis. Further study may show whether the concurrent administration of folinic acid has a significant ameliorating effect on the anemia of patients who have severe hemolysis. Folinic acid did not interfere with the therapeutic efficacy of pyrimethamine. Response to treatment was the same in patients treated with and without folinic acid. During the 30-day period of observation, there were no clinical or parasitologic recurrences in any of the patients studied.

I should like to illustrate two additional hematologic complications of malaria and their treatment by describing a case of recurrent falciparum malaria that lasted 6 months.

*Case report.* The patient was a 25-year-old white male who entered the Central Highlands of Vietnam in October 1966 (Figure 3). He received weekly Chloroquin-Primaquin tablets while there. One month after his arrival he developed fever, chills, headache, and muscular aches. A diagnosis of falciparum malaria was made by peripheral blood smear and the patient was hospitalized in early December. His initial treatment consisted of quinine 600 mg. every eight hours; pyrimethamine 25 mg. three times a day; and diaminodiphenylsulphone (DDS) 25 mg. daily. The pyrimethamine was given for three days and the quinine for three weeks. Despite this therapy and continued DDS, the patient again developed fever, and parasitemia in January, 1967. Between that recrudescence and his transfer to the Walter Reed Hospital, Washington D.C., the patient continued to have intermittent fever and parasitemia despite a variety of antimalarial programs. On one occasion therapy was interrupted because of pancytopenia, thought to be drug-induced. He was admitted to Walter Reed General Hospital on April 13, 1967. Physical examination at the time of admission showed a young Caucasian male who was febrile, pale, and icteric. The spleen was palpable 2 cm. below the left costal margin. A blood smear showed *P. falciparum.* The hematocrit was 18 per cent; white count 2,200 cells/mm.³; platelet count 100,000/mm.³; and the reticulocyte count was 7.8%. The serum bilirubin was 2.8 mg./100 ml. direct reacting fraction. Serum urea nitrogen was 35 mg./100 ml. Assay for red blood cell G-6-PD was normal. Urine urobilinogen was positive in 1:80 dilution. There was no significant urinary sediment. The patient had orthostatic hypotension, which improved after he received three units of whole blood. Two days after admission he developed a severe headache and his temperature increased to 103 degrees. He was given 600 mg. of quinine every eight hours; three units of blood were administered because of severe anemia. During the quinine therapy, the WBC count remained between 3,000 and 3,800 cells/mm.³ and the platelet count was 80 to 113,000/mm.³ Four additional units of blood were given because of continued hemolysis. On the fifth day of therapy the patient was afebrile and quinine was discontinued. The BUN had decreased to 13 mg./100 ml. Malaria smears were negative for two days, but again became positive on April 25 and the patient again became afebrile. A bone marrow examination obtained on April 28 showed erythrocytic hyperplasia with some dyspoiesis; granulocytic hypoplasia and malaria pigment were also present. Because of continued hemolysis and the lack of satisfactory response to previously administered antimalarial medication, trimethoprim 1,500 mg. daily was started on April 28 and was continued for seven days. After the fourth day of therapy, blood smears were negative for parasites and the patient was afebrile. During therapy the WBC count remained between 2,800 and 3,900 cells/mm.³ and the platelet count varied between 90,000 and 163,000/mm.³ Reticulocytes decreased from 13 to 1.5%. After five days of trimethoprim therapy, the bone marrow showed hypoplasia and megaloblastosis. After cessation of therapy, there was continued clinical improvement and all blood elements returned to normal.

Leukopenia occured on four occasions in this patient and coincided with recurrences of the infection and antimalarial therapy. Such a response is not usual. Decreased numbers of white cells in the peripheral blood is a common initial finding. However, with effective treatment, the white cell count increases and it is usually greater than 4,000 cells/mm.³ by the fourth day of therapy. This patient had a progressive decline in the count of white blood cells with therapy on at least three occasions. The bone marrow showed granulocytic hypoplasia. Other patients under similar circumstances have shown a maturation arrest of the myelocytic series. These finding may indicate an idiosyncratic reaction to one of the drugs employed.

This patient also had a severe hemolytic process while being treated with quinine for the last recurrence. Parasite density counts were low and did not account for the severe hemolysis. No evidence of a deficiency of glucose-6-phosphate dehydrogenase was found. The Coombs test was negative. However incubation of the patient's sera and normal red cells with quinine produced agglutination of the red blood cells (not observed with control sera). We therefore suspected that hemolysis in this patient was related to the administration of quinine and we treated him successfully with trimethoprim. The severe hemolytic episode occurred after prior courses of quinine not associated with comparable hemolysis. Quinine-associated hemolysis in patients from Vietnam had been seen previously after repeated courses of quinine. They have also shown a positive Coombs test.[18] The absence of a positive Coombs test in this patient suggests an unusual antigen-antibody reaction.

In summary, hematologic complications of malaria or malaria therapy include decreased circulating platelets, erythrocytes, and leukocytes. Thrombocytopenia is seen in association with consumptive coagulopathy or rarely in association with drug therapy. Severe hemolysis, although generally related to intense parasitemia, may be associated with specific red cell enzyme defects or with the administration of quinine. The usual patient with hemolysis secondary to malaria infections has a delayed erythropoietic response until parasitemia has been eradicated. Pyrimethamine probably does not contribute to the delayed response unless anemia is severe. Leukopenia is common during the first few days of an acute attack of malaria, but the count of white blood cells approaches normal with therapy. A decrease in circulating leukocytes to levels less than 3000/mm.[3] during therapy may represent an idiosyncratic reaction.

### REFERENCES

1. Sheehy, T. W., and Reba, R. C. Complications of falciparum malaria and their treatment. *Ann. Intern. Med. 66:* 807-09, 1967.

2. Blount, R. E., Jr. Acute falciparum malaria: Field experience with quinine/pyrimethamine combined therapy. *Ann. Intern, Med. 70:*142-47, 1969.

3. Brooks, M. H., Kiel, F. W. Sheehy, T. W. and Barry, K. G. Acute pulmonary edema in falciparum malaria: A clinicopathological correlation. *New Eng. J. Med. 279:*732-37, 1968.

4. Yamauchi, H. and Hanchett, J. E. *Acute Renal Failure Complicating South East Asia Falciparum Malaria* (abstract). Third International Congress of Nephrology, Sept. 25-30, 1966, Washington, D. C.

5. Canfield, C. J., Miller, L. H., Bartelloni, P. J. Eichler, P. and Barry, K. G. Acute renal failure in *Plasmodium falciparum* malaria, *Arch. Intern. Med. 122:*199-203, 1968.

6. Stone, W. J. and Knepshield, J. Acute renal insufficiency in falciparum malaria. In preparation.

7. Rosen, S. Hano, J. E., Inman, M. M., Gilliland, P. F. and Barry, K. G., The kidney in blackwater fever. *Amer. J. Clin. Path. 49*:358-70, 1968.

8. Donadio, J. V., Jr., and Whelton, A. Quinine therapy and peritoneal dialysis in acute renal failure complicating malarial haemoglobinuria. *Lancet 1:* 375-79, 1968.

9. Miller, L. H., Makaranond, P., Sitprija, V., Suebsanguan, C. and Canfield, C. J. Hyponatremia in malaria. *Ann. Trop. Med. Parasit. 61*:265-79, 1967.

10. Brooks, M. H., Malloy, J. P., Bartelloni, P. J., Tigertt, W. D., Sheehy, T. W. and Barry, K. G. Pathophysiology of acute falciparum malaria. *Amer. J. Med. 43*:735-50, 1967.

11. Dennis, L. H., Eichelberger, J. W., Inman, M. and Conrad, M. E. Depletion of coagulation factors in drug-resistant Plasmodium falciparum malaria. *Blood 27*:713-21, 1967.

12. Rosen, S. Mailloux, L. U., Lawson, N. J. and Teschan, P. E. Acute renal failure in the rat. *Lab. Invest. 18*:438-43, 1968.

13. Oken, D. E., Arce, M. L. and Wilson, D. R. Glycerol-induced hemoglobinuric acute renal failure in the rat. I. Micropuncture study of the development of oliguria. *J. Clin. Invest. 45*:724, 1966.

14. Cirksena, W. J., McNeil, J. and Gilliland, P. F. Personal communication.

15. Barry, K. G. and Crosby, W. H., The prevention and treatment of renal failure following transfusion reactions. *Transfusion 3*:34-36, 1963.

16. Conrad, M. E. Pathophysiology of malaria. *Ann. Intern. Med. 70*:134-41, 1969.

17. Canfield, C., Keller, H. and Cirksena, W. Erythrokinetics during treatment of acute falciparum malaria. In preparation.

18. Adner, M. M., Alstatt, L. B. and Conrad, M. E. Coombs'-positive hemolytic disease in malaria. *Ann. Intern. Med. 68*:33-38, 1968.

# CEREBRAL MALARIA*

HARRY MOST

Professor of Preventive Medicine
New York University School of Medicine
New York, N. Y.

THE term cerebral malaria has unfortunately conveyed to many clinicians the implication that the syndrome represents a severe infection with a virulent neurotropic strain of *P. falciparum*. Such a concept overlooks the severe systemic and organ involvements other than that in the nervous system and which in themselves may determine the course of the infection and its outcome. This concept is derived from the original clinical-pathological classification of the disease based on the predominant symptomatic manifestations such as cerebral, cardiovascular, renal, gastrointestinal, and hepatic types. My point is merely to emphsaize that all types exist simultaneously and vary only in degree. Appropriate treatment must recognize the diverse potential complications related to these systems as well as more recently appreciated problems such as defects of blood coagulation, the renal insufficiency syndrome, and even the possibility of autoimmune disease.

At this point it may be helpful for those of you who have not had occasion or reason to do so to review the principal lesions associated with severe falciparum infections. When this is done the clinical aspects are more readily understood and become apparent. Appreciation of the pathology also provides insight into the basis of rational therapy for the infection as a whole in addition to that intended to overcome major manifestations of the central nervous system.

A number of colored and of black and white lantern slides have been presented which have illustrated the major gross and microscopic lesions usually encountered in the brain, spleen, liver, kidney, bone marrow, and blood in fatal *P. falciparum* disease.

The brain appears pink to cherry red primarily because of the prominence of the vessels. The cut surfaces are similar in appearance, with a great contrast between the cortical gray and white matter which

*Presented as part of a *Symposium on Malaria* sponsored by The Tropical Disease Center, St. Clare's Hospital, New York, N. Y., and The Merck Company Foundation, Rahway, N. J., held at the Center, May 17, 1969.

has small vessels of larger caliber. Petechial hemorrhages may be widely distributed and especially noteworthy in the white matter. The gray matter may have a slate-blue cast because of the distended smaller veins.

The microscopic changes of greatest significance relate to the blood vessels, especially the capillaries. Many of these small vessels are occluded with parasitized red cells, free parasites, pigment, and red-cell debris. Other capillaries may be filled with plasma only, representing local spasm. Not infrequently aggregates of parasitized cells are found adhering to the endothelial lining, and in cross section of medium-sized vessels several layers of parasitized cells may be seen adjacent to the endothelial layer; the stream and center are free of parasites. Hemorrhages may be seen around and remote from small vessels, and they often present a ringlike appearance associated with dissolution of the enclosed brain material. Small granulomas or nodules composed of microglial cells that resemble lesions of typhus may also be seen.

The spleen is the organ most seriously affected; its role is often overlooked. The extensive pigmentation and the gross color of the spleen are due not only to the pigment of malaria but also to a marked reduction in the hyperemia. The parasitized cells are concentrated in the pulp. The follicles are depleted and there is considerable reduction in the number of lymphocytes, many of which have been transformed to macrophages. Appropriate staining will differentiate the pigments of iron and of malaria, which occur concomitantly.

The liver appears congested and the sinusoids exhibit dilatation. The Kupfer cells are increased in size and number and usually contain parasites or pigment. In severe infections there may also be extramedullary, periportal hematopoiesis. The bone marrow on the whole exhibits changes similar to that noted in the spleen, although fewer parasites are found than in the latter organ. There is evidence of marked phagocytosis of pigment and parasites. Characteristic changes are not related to any given form of anemia.

## CLINICAL ASPECTS

Stupor and coma of varying degree are the most prominent clinical manifestations of major cerebral involvement. Convulsions are frequent.

The neurological signs are neither consistent, localizing, nor specific. However the most common findings include stiffness of the neck, hyperreflexia, pyramidal tract signs, sucking and grasping reflexes, changing rigidities, and rectal and vesical incontinence. Rarely a cord-type bladder may be the only manifestation of impending severe cerebral involvement in a patient who is lucid and febrile with a high parasite count.

These neurological findings simply suggest an acute diffuse meningitic or encephalitic process. Unfortunately the spinal-fluid findings are not helpful in that the cells, globulin, chloride, etc., may not be altered and, if so, may vary in either direction.

The mental picture is one of confusion associated with restiveness, dullness, apathy, irritability, etc., and it provides no diagnostic clue to the underlying process.

It is evident from these brief remarks as well as the demonstration of the principal gross and microscopic findings that one must be alert to the systemic nature of severe falciparum disease; in its management one must not overlook one or more components which may lead to the patient's death despite control of the parasitemia and the principal, major clinical manifestation associated with the initial diagnosis.

# COMPLICATIONS OF FALCIPARUM MALARIA*

## BRIAN MAEGRAITH

Professor of Tropical Medicine
Liverpool School of Tropical Medicine
Liverpool, England

I PROPOSE to talk on the genesis and treatment of coma in malaria. The usual explanation given by pathologists for cerebral damage in falciparum malaria is the sometimes demonstrable "blocking" of the small vessels by parasitized erythrocytes. I am sure this is *post hoc* rather than *propter hoc* and is, in a sense, an artifact. It represents a late and usually irreversible development.

In my opinion the primary cause of coma is physiological barrier of the cerebral circulation. This is brought about by alteration of the function of the endothelial cells which are normally highly impermeable but which become permeable to protein (especially albumin) and so allow leakage of water. The protein and water leak into the contiguous brain tissue, where they cause some local edema, and into the cerebrospinal space through the blood-brain barrier. Since the villi are similarly disturbed, the protein passes freely back into the blood stream, so that the cerebrospinal fluid protein content becomes only moderately raised. This is quite different from the state of affairs in inflammatory meningitis, where protein can be shown to leak from the inflamed meningitic vessels but is *not* returned through the undisturbed villi; hence the cerebrospinal fluid protein content readily mounts.

The leakage of protein and of the accompanying water causes local increase in plasma viscosity and eventually stasis with packing of erythrocytes into a homogeneous mass which is essentially similar to that which occurs in vessels in acute inflammation.

The local circulation then slows and may come to a stop. I think it is this effect which finally induces coma in the patient.

The stasis is reversible for some time but eventually becomes irreversible, at which stage I suspect the balance of coagulation and fi-

*Presented as part of a *Symposium on Malaria* sponsored by The Tropical Disease Center, St. Clare's Hospital, New York, N.Y. and The Merck Company Foundation, Rahway, N.J., held at the Center, May 17, 1969.

brinolysis is tipped to the side of some intravascular clotting (which is seldom extensive and often not seen at all); this may be aggravated by "sludging."

This physiological picture occurs in many acute medical conditions, but in malaria it is complicated by the presence of the parasite and the specific effects it has on the host cell. The so-called plugging comes about because of the bursting of mature schizonts somewhere in the packed stased erythrocytes and high local infection rate caused by the merozoites.

If coma is due to the failing of the cerebral circulation, restoration of flow should be followed by recovery from coma. This is what I think happens immediately, but in the patient with malaria the ultimate outcome depends on two other factors: 1) the degree of irreversible damage which has occurred before therapy, and 2) the removal of the malaria parasites from the blood.

Thus in two comatose patients with severe falciparum malaria immediate treatment may restore consciousness in a few hours, but one patient may survive because the cerebral damage is largely reversible. This is independent of the rapid clearance of parasites in both cases.

Before I touch on the treatment of coma in malaria, let me summarize the experimental evidence for what I have said. We have demonstrated movement of albumin and water from cerebral vessels with the cerebral substance and the cerebrospinal fluid in both *Plasmodium berghei* and *Plasmodium knowlesi* infection, with the use of fluorescent, radioactive, and chemical and histochemical methods. We have demonstrated the edema by measuring dessicated brain weights and comparing the nitrogen and water content of samples of brain tissue. There is no doubt that the movement of protein and water occurs during the periods of high parasitemia.

We have also evidence of many factors in the circulation or at the tissue face which affect endothelial permeability in this way. Kininogens fall, kininogenases increase, kinin levels remain within normal limits despite a sometimes 10-fold increase in kininases; histamine and adenosine plasma levels rise. And so on—most of this has already been published, including the evidence of the existence of a toxic factor which inhibits oxidative phosphorylation in cell mitochondria, including those of endothelium.

Major support for the idea, however, comes also from treatment in the experimental model (and, as I see it, in falciparum malaria) once the escape of protein and water is stopped with extreme rapidity by cortisone and *by quinine and chloroquine.* All these compounds have very active anti-inflammatory actions, and here they act on the inflammatory stasis.

What is needed in the human case is an anti-inflammatory drug. We are lucky to have quinine and chloroquine which not only fulfill this requirement but are also antiparasitic.

In giving these drugs for cerebral malaria (let us say, for falciparum malaria) we are benefiting first by their anti-inflammatory activity and later by their antiparasitic action. In coma it is the former that counts, not the latter. This is obvious enough on the timing; recovery from coma after intravenous quinine occurs long before the drug has had time to act decisively on the parasite.

In most comatose cases that I have treated, I have found these drugs enough. I have not often felt justified in adding cortisone compounds, and I am not convinced that they are needed as a routine, as some advise.

Now a word about the pathogenesis and treatment of liver damage in infection from *Plasmodium falciparum.* All infections are associated with much evidence of liver damage, sometimes severe. The primary processes which initiate the hepatic disturbance are also sometimes associated with the onset of medical shock, sometimes not, but there is always considerable hyperactivity of the sympathetic nervous system. This is very clearly established in *P. knowlesi* malaria in macaque monkeys.

One effect of this is the constriction of visceral vessels and the resultant restriction of organ blood flows in the liver (and in the kidney). In the liver the small branches of the portal vein are most involved and the result of this constriction is portal venous hypertension and degeneration and necrosis of parenchymal cells in the centrilobular zones of the lobules, where the restricted blood flow and the inhibition of oxidative phosphorylation are additive.

We have found it possible in *P. knowlesi* malaria to release the portal venous constriction by adrenergic blockade. Ray produced a similar effect by sympathectomy before infection.

I suggest that in early hepatic failure in falciparum malaria it might be worth trying adrenergic blockade (for example by dibenzylene) which would not only relieve the circulating disturbances in the liver, but also in the vasconstricted kidney, in which acute anuric failure is not uncommon. (It is important to distinguish between the physiological circulating renal failure, which we demonstrated 25 years ago in blackwater fever, and the chronic renal lesions which appear in *Plasmodium* malariae infections, which probably have an immunological basis.)

I suppose what I am trying to say is: remember your physiology.

# PROPHYLACTIC CHEMOTHERAPY
# IN MALARIA*

JOHN D. ARNOLD

Professor of Medicine
Director, Harry S. Truman Medical Research Laboratory
University of Missouri
Kansas City, Mo.

E XCEPT for very rare cases of human infections acquired from monkeys, the chemoprophylaxis of malaria can be reduced to one of
two situations: 1) the chemotherapy of *Plasmodium falciparum* malaria
and 2) the chemotherapy of the relapsing malarias, such as *P. vivax*,
*P. ovale*, and *P. malariae*. Some understanding of the pathophysiology
of the malaria infection is relevant to the problems of chemotherapy
of malaria.

## *Plasmodium falciparum* MALARIA

In general *P. falciparum* infections are the hard core infections and
are eliminated last by eradication programs. Thus *P. falciparum* will be
with us for a long time. There is no known variation in racial resistance
in man, but the course of the disease varies from strain to strain of the
parasite. For instance, we have compared a strain from Uganda, Africa,
with the Camp strain from the Southwest Pacific. The Camp strain in
nonimmune subjects often produces a rising parasitemia which attains
a plateau at about 25,000 parasites/mm.[3] This is not true of a Uganda
strain, which may show an increase in parasite number until restrained
by the decreased numbers of circulating red cells. In experimental subjects the parasitemia produced by this strain has reached 600,000 para-
sites/mm.[3] with no indication of a halt without treatment.

The hazards of this disease are roughly correlated with the height
of the parasitemia.

Repeated infections with *P. falciparum* produce a form of immunity
that has sufficient force to moderate the course of new infections of the
same strain. This semi immune state has a very low mortality as com-

---

*Presented as part of a *Symposium on Malaria* sponsored by the Tropical Disease Center,
St. Clare's Hospital, New York, N.Y. and The Merck Company Foundation, Rahway, N.J., held
at the Center, May 17, 1969.
   This study was supported by U.S. Army Contract No. DA-49-193-MD-2545 from the U.S. Army
Research and Development Command, Office of the Surgeon General.

pared to the significant mortality seen in the nonimmune state. Thus the strategy of prophylactic chemotherapy may not be the same in nonimmunes as it is for semi-immunes.

The incubation period for *P. falciparum* is relatively short. Thus the chemotherapeutic agents which operate during the incubation period of five to seven days must be taken with great consistency because any drug failure however brief may allow merozoites to enter the red blood cell. After the red cells have been entered the disease presents an entirely new therapeutic challenge, for there seems to be little correlation between the causal prophylactic action of a drug and the suppressive action of a drug.

For this reason there is a tendency to classify antimalarial drugs according to the stage of the life cycle against which exerts its best action.[1] Thus a causal prophylactic agent works best against the tissue forms; this prevents parasitization of the blood cells. A suppressive cure should destroy blood forms. The prevention of red cell invasion by a suppressive drug is called clinical prophylaxis. Parasitization of the red cell and its consequences produces all the symptoms or signs of illness. In other words, the tissue forms of malaria are not known to produce illness.

In practice causal prophylaxis of *P. falciparum* malaria appears to be a very difficult objective. Very few agents have been developed that are capable of this effect. In fact, the same end result will come from long-acting suppressive agents and in *P. falciparum* malaria it is probably much safer to depend on suppressive cures than on an ideal prophylactic agent.

Even with the current distress about chloroquine resistance, we should remember that chloroquine when it works is a remarkably fine drug and is one which can be taken at intervals as great as once a week. Fortunately, the risk of encounter with a chloroquine-resistant strain of malaria can still be determined in part by geography. So far Africa is free of chloroquine-resistant *P. falciparum*. Table I shows the results of radical cure with chloroquine against a Uganda strain of *P. falciparum* from Africa in nonimmunes. Since these results in nonimmunes are consistent with the field experience with semi-immunes treated with chloroquine in Africa, it is not unreasonable to expect that 600 mg. of chloroquine will be a satisfactory treatment everywhere in Africa. Because chloroquine is excreted slowly and the parasitemia is slow to build

TABLE I.—THE CURATIVE RESPONSE OF A TYPICAL AFRICAN STRAIN OF *P. FALCIPARUM\** TO CHLOROQUINE IN NONIMMUNE SUBJECTS

| Dose of chloroquine | Ratio of cures to treated cases |
|---|---|
| 300 mg. | 4/8 |
| 450 mg. | 11/11 |
| 600 mg. | 2/2 |

\*The Uganda strain of *P. falciparum* malaria.

TABLE II.—THE CURATIVE RESPONSE OF CERTAIN CHLOROQUINE-RESISTANT STRAINS OF *P. FALCIPARUM* TO HIGH DOSES OF CHLOROQUINE

| Approximate curative dose of chloroquine | Origin of strain |
|---|---|
| 5.0 gm. | Brazil |
| > 4.0 gm. | Cambodia |
| > 3.0 gm. | Thailand |
| 3.0 gm. | Brazil |
| > 2.4 gm. | Venezuela |
| > 2.4 gm. | Columbia |
| > 1.5 gm. | Vietnam |

The symbol > indicates that cure requires a dose greater than that cited.

up from the tissue forms, this suppressive cure can be used on a once-weekly basis for prophylaxis. This 600-mg. dose is easily tolerated and therefore would seem to be preferable to the 450-mg. dose in the interest of greater certainty of protection for nonimmunes. However experience with the variation in dose response between strains is quite limited.

In some other parts of the world the problem is more difficult. Chloroquine resistance has been observed most often in Southeast Asia and South America. At present there does not exist a single satisfactory prophylactic agent for chloroquine-resistant *P. falciparum* malaria. As can be seen from Table II, a few selected experiences[2-8] with so-called chloroquine-resistant strains give a dosage that can approach serious toxicity. Since we have equated practical prophylaxis with suppressive cure, it is apparent that individuals on any practical regimen of chloroquine will run the risk of illness from *P. falciparum*.

Generally speaking, no precise measure of the ratio of incidence of

TABLE III.—COMPARISON OF RESPONSE OF A STRAIN OF *P. FALCIPARUM*
TO A SULFONAMIDE BEFORE AND AFTER INDUCED
PYRIMETHAMINE RESISTANCE

|  | *Sulfalene* | *Dose* | *Recurrence* |
|---|---|---|---|
| Before pryrimethamine resistance | 2.5 gm. | 1 time | 3/5 cases |
| After induced pryrimethamine resistance | 1.0 gm. | 1 time | 2/11 cases* |

*Recurrence in both cases was associated with loss of pyrimethamine resistance

resistant to nonresistant strains is available to us. Thus we can only guess at the degree of risk a given individual has of being exposed to drug-resistant malaria. It seems likely that certain strains will be chloroquine responsive, and that choloroquine will continue to have a prophylactic value in all parts of the world.

The problem of chloroquine resistance is under intense investigation at the moment; we can only offer some tentative suggestions for the prophylactic management of chloroquine resistance.

These suggestions are based on the early observations of Powell and Alving,[9] who reported a surprising degree of activity of diamino diphenyl sulfone in chloroquine-resistant *P. falciparum* infections.

The activity of the sulfones and sulfonamides has not always been considered very important. In the past the value of sulfonamides has been regarded as uncertain. Coggeshall et al.[10] found that in five patients treated with sulfadiazine two infections were unchanged by the drug and, in three infections, the parasites were eliminated.

This study with others was sufficient to lessen the enthusiasm for sulfonamides. An explanation for the variability in response of *P. falciparum* to sulfones and sulfonamides is suggested by recent studies in human volunteers. These studies are reviewed in Table III.[11] In brief they show that normal strains tend to be poorly responsive to sulfonamides. After the strain is made resistant to pyrimethamine the response to sulfonamide is greatly improved. In a nonpyrimethamine-resistant group a dose of 2.5 gm. gave a cure in only two of five subjects. In a pyrimethamine-resistant group, a dose of 1 gm. cured 9 of 11 subjects. In the first instance, the rate of parasite clearance was slow and, in the second instance, the rate of parasite clearance was rapid. The two failures in the pyrimethamine group were shown on reexamination to be

TABLE IV.—A COMPARISON OF RESPONSE BETWEEN A NORMAL STRAIN OF *P. FALCIPARUM* (UGANDA) AND A PYRIMETHAMINE-RESISTANT STRAIN OF *P. FALCIPARUM* (CAMP)

| Sulfalene | Uganda recurrences | Camp recurrences |
|---|---|---|
| 1 gm. | 3/5 | 0/10 |
| 2.5 gm. | 3/6 | — |

TABLE V.—THE CONCURRENCE OF PYRIMETHAMINE RESISTANCE IN STRAINS ALSO CHLOROQUINE-RESISTANT FROM REPORTS IN THE LITERATURE

|  | Pyrimethamine | Chloroquine |
|---|---|---|
| Malayan Camp | > 150 mg. | > 3.0 gm. |
| Thailand (AND) | > 150 mg. | > 1.5 gm. |
| Vietnam (CV) | > 150 mg. | > 1.5 gm. |
| Goiania (Brazil) | > 300 mg. | 8.0 gm. |
| Para I (Brazil) | > 0.30 mg. | > 2.4 gm. |
| Columbian III | > 0.30 mg. | > 2.4 gm. |

strains which had lost their pyrimethamine resistance.

There is little reason to suspect that there is any great qualitative difference in the sulfonamides or sulfones for that matter, as long as dose and duration of treatment are adequate. Recent studies in our laboratory showed that for suppressive cure of a sensitive strain, a sulfonamide should have a duration of action for at least three days.

A comparison of strain responses isolated from the field is available from a comparison of the Camp and Uganda strains. In Table IV[12] we see that the pyrimethamine-resistant Camp strain is quite sensitive to sulfalene as compared to the normal Uganda strain. In this study these two strains closely resemble the counterpart experience with the Uganda strain and the induced pyrimethamine resistant Uganda. Often we see a marked tendency for resistance to one drug, chloroquine, to be associated with resistance to the other drug, pyrimethamine (Table V).[13]

The finding that resistance to one drug, pyrimethamine, reduces the dose requirement for another drug, sulfalene, raises some interesting questions about mechanisms of drug action. For example, the metabolism of the parasite may be placed between the metabolism of two great groups of organisms. On the one hand, the bacteria which synthesize

73

TABLE VI.—THE MOST VULNERABLE POINT OF DRUG ATTACK

*In strains with pyrimethamine resistance*
↓
PABA ⇸ folic Acid ⇸ folinic Acid
*In strains which are not pyrimethamine resistant*

Sulfonamides

pyrimethamine*
↓
PABA ⇸ folic Acid ⇸ folinic Acid

*And other folic acid reductase inhibitors such as chloroguamide and trimethoprim.

folic acid and, on the other hand, higher animals including man, who absorb folic acid and are often sensitive to folic acid reductase inhibitors. The parasite is most dependent on folic acid synthesis when it is resistant to a reductase inhibitor. It thus resembles the bacteria. When it is not resistant to pyrimethamine, it is only partially dependent on folic acid synthesis and it somewhat resembles higher organisms.

These findings would also alter the interpretation of the often discussed synergism between sulfonamide and pyrimethamine.[14] The argument, as most frequently stated, attributes this synergism to a sequential block at two points of folic acid metabolism in the same organism (Table VI). Rather, it would seem that a given organism can be sensitive either to the inhibition of para-aminobenzoic acid or reductase. Synergism in this case would be due to the fact that only one of the two groups of organisms is affected by a given drug. The other strain is affected by the other drug.

I have strayed into a discussion of suppressive cures because I believe that a practical causal prophylactic agent against *P. falciparum* malaria must also be effective against the circulating trophozoite. There are a number of other agents for suppressive cure: quinine and trimethoprim alone, quinine in combination with pyrimethamine and the sulfonamides or sulfone. At present their use is limited to the treatment of acute attacks, because they do not have a long duration of action. Sulfone given daily can reduce the attack rate of chloroquine-resistant *P. falciparum;* it is currently in use in Vietnam.

In summary, it should be reemphasized that chloroquine is still the drug of choice for prophylaxis of *P. falciparum* infection. In those areas of the world where chloroquine resistance has appeared, chloroquine should be used with a sulfone or sulfonamide. Very recently progress

Table VII.—RELATION BETWEEN CURATIVE DOSE OF PYRIMETHAMINE
AND THE NUMBER OF PARASITES IN PERIPHERAL BLOOD

| Dose of pyrimethamine | Highest observed parasite count/mm.³ | | | |
|---|---|---|---|---|
| | $< 1,000$ | 1,000 to 20,000 | 20,000 to 100,000 | $> 200,000$ |
| 12.5 mg. | 3/5* | 0/1 | | |
| 25.0 mg. | 10/10 | 0/5 | | |
| 50.0 mg. | | | 0/2 | |
| 100.0 mg. | | | | 0/1 |

*Ratio of cure to treatment.

has been made by the Army in developing an oral long-acting sulfone. At this point in time, it would appear that failures would be reduced though probably not eliminated by using any of these agents. The reason for a limited number of failures in prophylaxis where a combination of chloroquine and folic acid synthetase inhibitor was used has not yet been analyzed.

### Plasamodium vivax MALARIA

This malaria is the classic relapsing form; it exists in two varieties, depending on the relapse pattern. These two forms are compared in a schematic way with each other and with *falciparium malaria* in Table VIII. These differences are of some practical importance. In the case of the late relapsing form, the first relapse or even the first acute attack may occur as long as nine months after the subject has left an endemic zone. In general these late relapses will not occur with the quick relapsing P. *vivax* and they should never occur with P. *falciparum*.

For the most part, the quick relapsing P. *vivax* malarias have been encountered in the southwest Pacific area and Southeast Asia. The late relapsing forms of P. *vivax* infection have been reported from Europe, Korea, Madagascar, and the United States. This suggests that these forms have been adapted to more temperate zones and that the late relapse has the effect of keeping the infection dormant over winter.

P. *vivax* is also different from P. *falciparum* in that there is a very substantial difference in susceptibility toward the infection; this depends on the race of the patient. It is well documented that pure-blooded Negroes are virtually immune to P. *vivax* and that many patients with mixed Negro and white ancestry show intermediate degrees of resis-

75

tance. As a consequence the risk of infection to *P. vivax* and the consequent need for prophylaxis can be estimated in part by the ethnic character of the region from which the exposure is experienced.

In Haiti, for instance, *P. vivax* is rare; *P. falciparum* is common. *P. vivax* is rare or absent from West Africa.

The destruction of the late tissue forms of either quick or late relapsing *P. vivax* is often termed a radical cure. It is fortunate that *P. vivax* infections are not threatening to life. Thus failure of a drug used in causal prophylaxis will not be disastrous. In addition one may hope that the relapse pattern will terminate spontaneously at the end of the second year. Thus the major benefit to be derived from prophylaxis is freedom from illness for a period of about two years.

The primary problem of prophylaxis in this form of malaria is the destruction of the tissue stages. A drug effective against the tissue stages will terminate the relapse pattern. Unfortunately such drugs as chloroquine and quinine, which are effective against the blood stages of *P. vivax*, as well as of *P. falciparum*, are quite ineffective against the tissue stages.

At this time there appear to be only two classes of drug which have demonstrated an action against the tissue stages of *P. vivax* malaria in man. One class of drugs is the 8-amino quinolines, which have a chemical history dating back to methylene blue. The other class of drug are the folic acid reductase inhibitors of which pyrimethamine is the prototype.

Some authorities wait for evidence of infection before instituting a course of primaquine prophylaxis against the secondary tissue stages. If the risk of infection in a given individual is slight, there may be merit in this approach. Though the discomfort of acute malaria may be great, the danger of an attack of *P. vivax* infection is very small. Drug toxicity may be substantial and thus may justify a calculated gamble.

The patient may take 30 to 45 mg. of primaquine once or twice weekly for 8 weeks, or a weekly program may be maintained continuously during the entire stay in an endemic zone. In either case, chloroquine is given simultaneously to cover the risk of a parasite breakthrough. This approach has been instituted by the military services during the war in Vietnam.

A continuous 14 day course of once daily primaquine (15 mg.) and chloroquine may be used. This program probably achieves the best therapeutic results, but it does require a cooperative patient or a controlled group of patients. This program was used with considerable effect during the Korean War.[15] In that situation, troops who were known to have a significant incidence of latent infection with a late relapsing form of *P. vivax* were available for 10 to 14 days during the trip back to the United States by ship. A substantial reduction of the incidence of *P. vivax* malaria was reported to have followed this program.

Not all studies on the efficacy of primaquine prophylaxis agree. Some general conclusions, however, seem possible: the usual experience with any regimen of primaquine, at doses less than those that produce considerable toxicity, is for failure rates to vary between 5% and 20%.

There is a suggestion from various data that the number of sporozoites inoculated accounts for part of these differences. A heavy inoculum means a lower rate of protection for a given dose. This was noticed in the early studies done during World War II with a variety of 8-amino-quinoline. When the mosquito inoculum fell below a certain arbitrary point, the cure rate of a given drug was much higher than if the inoculum were above this arbitrary level.

Another reason for a less than perfect protection rate is related to the problem of administering 8 or 14 doses of drug without fail. This is more than one can reasonably expect in a large group of subjects. It should be remembered that the drug is being pushed to its maximum effect under the most favorable circumstances and that any reduction below the optimal dose will inevitably reduce the therapeutic efficacy.

A discussion of primaquine probably requires a word about toxicity.

There may be a sizable amount of gastrointestinal distress of a degree sufficient to make some people stop taking the drug. The extent of this distress has not been measured accurately and has been the subject of controversy. Nevertheless, after long personal experience with this drug, I believe that some patients are adversely affected.

There is a real incidence of mild self-limited hemolytic anemia, caused for the most part by deficiency of glucose-6-phosphate dehydrogenase.

Many reviews have been written about the toxic effect of primaquine on the red blood cell; this information is readily accessible.[16] Suffice it to say that primaquine-induced hemolysis opened the way for

TABLE VIII.—THREE TYPES OF MALARIA

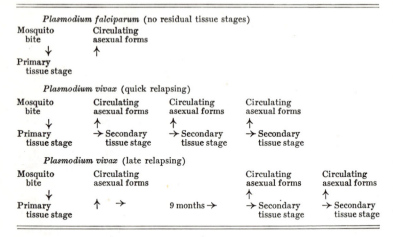

the elucidation of a series of inherited enzyme deficiencies of the red cell. The Negro patient, who has great inherent resistance to *P. vivax* malaria and thus has less need for primaquine, however, is most often affected with primaquine-induced hemolysis.

This becomes a practical problem of some consequence only when one cannot withhold primaquine from patients on the basis of race. Fortunately the sensitive red cells are usually the old red cells. When these have been hemolyzed, the young replacement red cells are relatively invulnerable and the anemia decreases though administration of the drug is continued. This self-limited aspect of primaquine hemolysis in patients who have glucose-6-phosphate deficiency has made the problem much less serious than might have been expected.

While primaquine has been the most intensively studied causal prophylactic, it is also certain that pyrimethamine, chlorguanide, and other folic acid reductase inhibitors, such as trimethoprim, may share this property.

The major difficulty attending the use of pyrimethamine and chlorguanide is the ease with which they induce drug resistance. It does not seem to matter how large a dose is used. If the surviving parasites are not killed, they will show resistance to almost any tolerated dose of pyrimethamine. Here again we encounter a relation between the number of parasites and the dose of a drug required for cure. A dramatic relation appears to exist between the number of parasites and the curative dose. This is shown in Table VII.[17] At high parasitemias a maximum dose of pyrimethamine may fail to cure.

## *Plasmodium ovale* and *Plasmodium malariae* MALARIAS

*P. ovale* is the relapsing malaria of West Africa. From the very limited information available, this parasite appears to have a short life span, much as *P. vivax* does; probably it responds to the same drugs that cure *P. vivax* infections.

*P. malariae* (quartan malaria), on the other hand, may produce relapses over many years. Not only has the drug response of this species received very little attention, but it will be very difficult to measure the effectiveness of the anti-relapse or causal prophylactic action of a drug against quartan malaria because of the enormous span of time during which the infection must be observed. At this time it would seem reasonable to treat quartan malaria as if it were *P. vivax* and hope for the best.

### SUMMARY

A practical prophylactic agent in *P. falciparum* malaria should also destroy schizonts in the blood. Such a drug is chloroquine and it should probably always be used once a week by persons in areas where *P. falciparum* is endemic even though resistant strains are known to be present. In Africa the single weekly dose should be at least 600 mg. of chloroquine base.

In areas of possible cloroquine resistance, this program should be supplemented by a sulfone or sulfonamide. In doses equivalent to 2 gm. sulfadiazine per day for 3 days in one week, these drugs will protect against many chloroquine-resistant strains. The sulfone or sulfonamide may be long acting or may be given once daily. It is difficult to be more specific about doses because investigation of these compounds is not complete.

Although casual prophylaxis of *P. vivax* is still relatively unsatisfactory, a 10- to 14-day course of treatment with primaquine, or a weekly dose for 8 weeks with doses of 30 to 45 mg. will reduce sharply the risk of relapse. A somewhat more satisfactory cure rate will probably result from 14 days of continuous therapy with 15 mg. to 25 mg. daily, but this is often harder to manage.

Causal prophylaxis against *P. vivax* should be accompanied by chloroquine to protect against errors in drug administration.

## ACKNOWLEDGMENTS

We thank Sheriff Kenneth Carnes and his staff for their cooperation in these studies. We are especially grateful to the inmate volunteers from the Jackson County Jail, Kansas City, Mo., whose cooperation made this study possible.

*REFERENCES*

1. Bruce-Chwatt, L. J. Classification of anti-malarial drugs in relation to different stages in the life cycle of the parasite: Commentary on a diagram. *Bull. WHO 27*:287-90, 1962.
2. Martin, D. C. and Arnold, J. D. Studies on an East African Strain of *Plasmodium falciparum. Trans. Roy. Soc. Trop. Med. Hyg. 61*:331-39, 1965.
3. Montgomery, R. and Eyles, D. E. Chloroquine resistant falciparum malaria in Malaya. *Trans. Roy. Soc. Trop. Med. Hyg. 57*:409-16, 1963.
4. Moore, D. V. and Lanier, J. E. Observations on two *Plasmodium falciparum* infections with an abnormal response to chloroquine. *Amer. J. Trop. Med. 10*:5-9, 1961.
5. Powell, R. D., Brewer, G. J., Alving, A. F. and Millar, J. W. Studies on a strain of chloroquine-resistant *Plasmodium falciparum* from Thailand. *Bull. WHO 30*:29-44, 1964.
6. WHO Scientific Group. Resistance of malaria parasites to drugs. *WHO Techn. Rep. 296*, 1965.
7. Young, M. D. and Moore, D. V. Chloroquine resistance in *Plasmodium falciparum. Amer. J. Trop. Med. 10*:317-320, 1961.
8. Walker, A. J. Personal communication, 1965.
9. Powell, R. D. et al. *Op. cit.*, pp. 29-44.
10. Coggeshall, L. T., Maier, J. and Best, C. A. The effectiveness of two new types of chemotherapeutic agents in malaria. *J.A.M.A. 117*:1077-81, 1941.
11. Martin, D. C. and Arnold, J. D. Enhanced sensitivity of *P. falciparum* to sulfalene as a consequence of resistance to pyrimethamine. *Trans. Roy. Soc. Trop. Med. Hyg.* In press.
12. Martin, D. C. and Arnold, J. D. The drug response of a normal and a multiresistant strain of *P. falciparum* to sulphalene. *Trans. Roy. Soc. Trop. Med. Hyg. 62*:810-815, 1968.
13. Martin, D. C. and Arnold, J. D. *Op. cit.* (ref. 2), pp. 337-38.
14. Alving, A. S., Arnold, J. and Robinson, D. H. Status of primaquine. 1. Mass therapy of subclinical vivax malaria with primaquine. *J.A.M.A. 149*:1558-62, 1952.
15. Alving, A. S. et al., Ibid.
16. Carson, P. E. and Tarlov, A. R. Biochemistry of hemolysis. *Ann. Rev. Med. 13*:105-26, 1962.
17. Martin, D. C. and Arnold, J. D. The effect of parasite populations on the curative action of pyrimethamine. *Trans. Roy. Soc. Trop. Med. Hyg. 62*:379-84, 1968.

# TREATMENT OF MALARIA INFECTION*

## Peter G. Contacos

Head, Section on Primate Malaria
National Institutes of Allergy and Infectious Diseases
Atlanta-Chamblee, Ga.

MANY drugs are available for the specific treatment of malaria. For clinical use these are divided into those which act primarily on the erythrocytic asexual stages (blood schizonticides) and those which act primarily on the tissue (liver) stages (tissue schizonticides). Drugs that act on the erythrocytic asexual stages effect only clinical cures in the case of relapsing malarias (vivax, malariae, and ovale). In the case of falciparum malaria, which does not have residual or persisting tissue stages and therefore does not relapse, blood schizonticides alone can effect radical cure. Drugs which act upon the tissue stages can effect radical cures of relapsing malaria when used in conjunction with an effective blood schizonticide.

Quinine, an alkaloid of cinchona bark, has been used as an antimalarial agent for more than 3 centuries. Quinacrine (Atabrine) was introduced in 1930, chloroquine (Aralen) and chlorguanide (Paludrine) in 1945, amodiaquine (Camoquin) in 1948, and pyrimethamine (Daraprim) in 1950. Each of these drugs is a blood schizonticide and all except quinine are synthetic compounds. In addition there are two synthetic 8-aminoquinoline compounds, pamaquine and primaquine, which are used clinically for the radical treatment of relapsing malarias because they act primarily on the tissue stages.

Of all the synthetic antimalarial drugs available for the treatment of clinical attacks of drug-sensitive malaria, chloroquine remains the favorite. However, because availability of drugs differs in various areas, the recommended dosage regimens for all the antimalarials will be reviewed.

Quinine is available in the form of 2 salts. Quinine sulfate in the form of 5 gr. (0.325 gm.) tablets or capsules is most often administered for oral therapy. A total dosage of 210 gr. (13.65 gm.) is given as follows:

---

*Presented as part of a *Symposium on Malaria* sponsored by The Tropical Disease Center, St. Clare's Hospital, New York, N.Y. and The Merck Company Foundation, Rahway, N.J., held at the Center, May 17, 1969.

10 gr. (0.65 gm.) every eight hours for seven days. Quinine dihydro-chloride is available when parenteral administration is required for emergency use. No more than 0.65 gm. (10 gr.) dissolved in 20 ml. of sterile diluent should be given in any six- to eight-hour period. Intravenous quinine must be given very slowly. Because rapid intravenous administration of quinine is hazardous, it is recommended that it be given, when required, as a slow intravenous infusion using 10 gr. of quinine in 500 ml. of sterile saline. Quinine can terminate acute attacks of all the malarias and radically cure falciparum malaria sensitive to it.

Quinacrine (Atabrine, Mepacrine) is available in 100 mg. tablets as quinacrine hydrochloride. The recommended dosage regimen is a total of 2.8 gm. given over a period of 7 days as follows: 200 mg. (2 tablets) every 6 hours for 5 doses (loading dose) followed by 100 mg. (1 tablet) every 8 hours for 6 days. Because the 4-aminoquinolines are less toxic, more efficacious, and easier to administer, they (chloroquine, amodiaquine) are preferred over quinacrine.

Chlorguanide (Paludrine, proguanil) is available in 100-mg. tablets as the hydrochloride. The therapeutic regimen consists of a total dosage of 1.5 gm. given as follows: 100 mg. every 8 hours for 5 days. Because of its slow action in acute clinical attacks, it is not generally recommended over the 4-aminoquinolines. This drug has the tendency to produce resistance when given in subcurative dosages.

Pyrimethamine (Daraprim) is available in 25-mg. tablets of the base. A single dose of 50 mg. (2 tablets) can terminate an attack of malaria but because of its slow action it is not recommended for treatment of acute attacks. This drug, like chlorguanide, also has the tendency to produce resistance.

Chloroquine (Aralen) is available in the form of 250-mg. tablets of chloroquine diphosphate, each tablet containing 150 mg. of the base. The therapeutic oral regimen of chloroquine is a total dosage of 1.5 gm. of the *base* given as follows: 600 mg. (4 tablets) at once, followed by 300 mg. (2 tablets) at 6, 24, and 48 hours after the first dose. When parenteral therapy is indicated, as in the case of coma or with protracted nausea and vomiting, chloroquine dihydrochloride is available in 10-ml. ampules containing approximately 450 mg. of the salt or 400 mg. of the active base. The contents of the ampule (10 ml.) can be given by injecting 5 ml. intramuscularly in each buttock. Chloroquine may be given intravenously. However intravenous use, in my opinion, should not be necessary since effective chloroquine levels obtain within 15 minutes after intramuscular injection which is approximately the time that would be required to give this amount of chloroquine intravenously.

Amodiaquine (Camoquin), a synthetic 4-aminoquinoline, like chloroquine, is available as tablets of amodiaquine dihydrochloride dihydrate containing 200 mg. active base. The dosage regimen is 600 mg. base (3 tablets) at once followed by 400 mg. base (2 tablets) at 24 and 48 hours. There are no significant advantages in using this drug over chloroquine.

Primaquine, a synthetic 8-aminoquinoline, is available as 26.3-mg. tablets of the phosphate salt containing 15-mg. base. Since chloroquine and the other drugs already mentioned have no appreciable effect if any against the tissue stages responsible for relapses of vivax, malariae, and ovale malaria, cures for these malarias cannot be obtained by treatment with these drugs alone. Complementary therapy with primaquine is required. The dosage regimen for radical cure of the relapsing malarias is as follows: 1 tablet (15-mg. base) daily for 14 consecutive days.

When resistance of parasites is not suspected, chloroquine or another 4-aminoquinoline is considered the treatment of choice for termination of the acute attack of all four human malarias. In falciparum malaria which, so far as is known, does not relapse, treatment with chloroquine alone results in radical cure. However, in vivax, malariae, and ovale malarias, all of which are considered to be relapsing malarias, complementary therapy with primaquine must be given to achieve radical cure. It should be pointed out that, with some strains of vivax malaria, one can expect a failure rate of up to 30% with the 14-day regimen of primaquine.

Unfortunately we cannot end our discussion on the subject of the chemotherapy of clinical malaria at this point. This is primarily because of the appearance of falciparum malaria resistant to chloroquine, the compound which had attained worldwide acceptance as the antimalarial of choice because of its proved efficacy during many years of use. Resistance of falciparum parasites to chloroquine was first observed in September of 1960 by Moore and Lanier and reported by them in 1961 in patients who had been in Colombia, South America.[1] Since then, resistant strains of falciparum malaria have been reported and documented from Brazil, Thailand, Cambodia, Malaysia, and South Vietnam.

The full extent of the problem in most of these areas is not known. Reports from these areas indicate that from 20% up to as high as 90% of the strains or cases of falciparum malaria are resistant to some antimalarial agent. We must keep in mind that for the time being most of the strains resistant to chloroquine are of the R-I or R-II types as defined by the WHO Study Group on Chemotherapy[2] (R-I): clearance of asexual parasitemia followed by recrudescence; R-II: marked reduction of asexual parasitemia but without clearance.

As stated earlier the treatment of falciparum malaria sensitive to chloroquine is relatively simple and straightforward, i.e., the 1.5-gm. regimen of chloroquine base given in a 48-hour period is curative.

The treatment of chloroquine-resistant falciparum, however, is another story. Early in the days of resistance to chloroquine, the one drug that was found to cure multiresistant malaria consistently was quinine; and for this reason whenever chloroquine-resistance was evident, the treatment of choice was quinine sulfate (10 gr. every 8 hours for 5 to 7 days). Resistance to chloroquine should be suspected when a patient gives a history of having returned from an area where chloroquine-resistant strains are prevalent *and*, in addition, suppressive chloroquine was taken in the endemic area as well as for at least several weeks after departure from the area.

There were actually no serious problems with the treatment of chloroquine-resistant falciparum malarias until about 1964, when strains principally from South Vietnam were found to be resistant to dosages of quinine previously known to be radically curative not only for chloroquine-sensitive strains but also for the chloroquine-resistant strains from South America and other countries in Southeast Asia.

Obviously these reports of falciparum parasites resistant in varying degrees to all known acceptable antimalarial drugs including quinine indicated a pressing need for alternative regimens. Although in the past 5 years or so, there have been many reports concerned with the evaluation of various alternative regimens for the treatment of multiresistant falciparum malaria, only some of them will be summarized here. These methods consist of combinations of two or three drugs, one or two of which always constitutes a known standard antimalarial. Usually, the second or third agent has been a sulfonamide or sulfone.

I hesitate to discuss or review many of the alternative regimens which have been described for the treatment of multiresistant falciparum malarias, especially from Southeast Asia. I hesitate primarily because from the point of view of the civilian physician, many of the compounds in this alternative methods either have not been licensed by the Food and Drug Administration for general use in this country or are not readily available through local pharmacies throughout the country.

### Sulfonamides Combined with Pyrimethamine

Initially the search for alternative regimens involved a reevaluation of sulfonamides and sulfones alone and in combination with pyrimethamine. These compounds had been shown to have some antimalarial effect in the early 1940's but were shelved because of the development of other more effective antimalarial agents such as chloroquine. In addition, potentiation effects had been reported[3-5] for combinations of pyrimethamine with sulfonamides or with sulfone (diaminodiphenylsulfone, DDS, Dapsone).

The most promising regimen under this combination is Fanzil (sulphormethoxine) 1 gm. with 50 mg. of pyrimethamine given as a single dose.[6-8] This combination has given an almost 100% radical curative rate when administered for primary attacks of chloroquine-resistant falciparum malaria in nonimmune patients. Other sulfonamides such as sulfadiazine or Midicel can be substituted for Fanzil but these would have to be given at conventional doses for a minimum of five days.

Toxicity of some of the long-acting sulfonamides has been one of the reasons for caution in the use of such compounds, although in the single dose of 1 gm. this is not considered a serious problem. Rather we were, and in fact still are, of the opinion that the chief limitation to the large scale use of sulfonamides as antimalarials is the ease with which resistance can be developed by malaria parasites and other microorganisms to this class of compounds.

### Sulfones

Most of the studies with sulfones have indicated that these substances would be useful more as suppressive than as therapeutic agents;[9,10] i.e., DDS alone would not be satisfactory for the treatment of acute attacks of malaria. Although the principal use of sulfones (Dapsone) in troops in South Vietnam is that of a suppressive, it is also being used therapeutically to supplement various combination regimens.[11-13] When various alternative regimens such as quinine-pyrimethamine or chloroquine-quinine were supplemented by the administration of 25 mg. of Dapsone for a period of 28 to 30 days during convalescence or following the completion of the combined therapy, recrudescence rates were reduced from 50% to 5% or less. One group of authors,[13] in recognition of the fact that dapsone is not available to civilians at present, indicated that sulfadiazine (0.5 gm. every 6 hours for 5 days) could be substituted for Dapsone.

## QUININE SULFATE ALONE OR IN COMBINATIONS

Quinine sulfate has probably been the antimalarial most consistently used for the treatment of acute attacks of chloroquine-resistant falciparum malaria in Vietnam, whether alone or in combination with one or more other drugs. Legters[14] in 1965 suggested that quinine (30 gr. daily for 10 days) was probably the best drug available at that time for termination of acute attacks of chloroquine-resistant falciparum malaria. Although he suggested that concurrent administration of pyrimethamine and sulfadiazine given after termination of the acute attack by quinine sulfate might increase the radical curative rate, he did not recommend concurrent administration of pyrimethamine and sulfadiazine alone for treatment of acute attacks. Blount[15] reported that quinine sulfate (600 mg. every 8 hours for 14 days) and pyrimethamine (25 mg. every 12 hours for 3 days) given to approximately 2,000 cases of acute falciparum malaria resulted in good clinical and parasitologic response in all cases.

## COMBINATION OF TWO NEW COMPOUNDS, SULFALENE AND TRIMETHOPRIM

The most recent combination of drugs proposed as an alternative for the treatment of acute falciparum malaria is the combination of sulfalene, a long-acting sulfonamide, and a dihydrofolic acid reductase inhibitor, trimethoprim. Martin and Arnold[16] reported that the combination was able to cure eight of eight patients with ordinary falciparum malaria (0.25 gm. sulfalene and 0.125 gm. trimethoprim as a single dose) and 10 of 11 patients with multiresistant falciparum malaria (0.75 gm. sulfalene and 0.5 gm. trimethoprim). To me, the one outstanding feature of this combination is its apparent ability to clear parasites and lyse fever rapidly in drug-sensitive as well as drug-resistant strains of falciparum malaria. A rapid clinical response with many of the other combinations is not observed consistently. It has recently been observed, however, that this combination of drugs does not have the same excellent results against all strains of falciparum upon which it has been tried.

It is obvious from the foregoing review that there are many alternative therapeutic regimens for use against falciparum infections that exhibit resistance not only to chloroquine and other synthetic antimalarial agents but also to quinine. In Vietnam the current treatment of choice for falciparum malaria is the combination of quinine sulfate, pyrimethamine, and Dapsone. The radical curative rate for this regimen is estimated to be approximately 95%. Even with the availability of these alternative methods some have continued to recommend the initial use of quinine alone in the treatment of acute attacks of suspected chloroquine-resistant falciparum malaria in nonimmune individuals and to keep one of the alternative combinations for patients whose infections recrudesce after adequate quinine therapy (10 gr. every 8 hours for at least 7 days).

For many reasons I agree with this opinion. Many of the combinations, especially of the pyrimethamine and sulfonamide types, have generally not effected rapid clinical response even though they can effect radical cure. On the other hand, quinine has usually effected good clinical response and at least temporary clearance of parasitemia even in persons infected with falciparum malaria resistant to quinine. There are also some infections which show good clinical response but only minimal parasitologic response. Where there is a recrudescence of parasitemia after adequate quinine therapy or in cases where adequate response is not observed in 24 hours, or in cases where idiosyncratic response to quinine is observed, the course is obvious: one of the alternative regimens should be adopted.

A major reason for my preference to achieve radical cure with quinine alone if this is possible without endangering the patient and for my preference for one of the alternative methods only after the failure of quinine, is the fact that most of the combinations include drugs which belong to a class of compounds to which microorganisms easily develop resistance. Even in the combinations where a potentiation effect is evident, this potentiation could become ineffective if the degree of resistance to one or both of the drugs increases. Some of our observations in studies with the injectable mixture known as CI-564 indicate that this phenomenon can occur with ease.[17] Whereas the combination of Fanzil and pyrimethamine effected radical cure in 11 of 11 patients infected with two strains of falciparum malaria (resistant to chloroquine, chlorguanide, pyrimethamine, and quinacrine), this same combination failed to effect a radical cure in four of five patients whose infections with these same two strains were not cured by CI-564, which is a sulfone-and-chlorguanide type compound. In other words, increased cross resistance to the combination of Fanzil and pyrimethamine obtained through a single prior exposure of these two strains of falciparum malaria parasites to a sulfone or chlorguanide compound.

Because of all the problems associated with the treatment of falciparum malarias, I believe that hospitalization should be recommended so that such patients can be carefully supervised and their progress followed by blood smears for parasite counts at least every 12 hours. It should also be pointed out that the physician's responsibility does not end with the treatment. The patient should be followed for 90 days.

Finally, we must remember in treating falciparum malaria today that, irrespective of the therapeutic regimen used, we can at present no longer be certain of a radical cure until a compound proved to be 100% effective is again available. The need for new compounds is obvious.

### REFERENCES

1. Moore, D. and Lanier, J. Observations on two *Plasmodium falciparum* infections with an abnormal response to chloroquine. *Amer. J. Trop. Med. 10:*5, 1961.
2. WHO *Chemotherapy of Malaria.* Techn. Rep. 375. Geneva, WHO, 1967.
3. Rollo, I. The mode of action of sulphonamides, proguanil, and pyrimethamine on *Plasmodium gallinaceum. Brit. J. Pharmacol. 10:*208, 1955.
4. Hurly, M. Potentiation of pyrimethamine by sulphadiazine in human malaria. *Trans. Roy. Soc. Trop. Med. Hyg. 53:*412, 1959.
5. Basu, P., Singh, N. N. and Singh, N. Potentiation of activity of diaphenylsulfone and pyrimethamine against *Plasmodium gallinaceum* and *Plasmodium cynomolgi bastianellii.* Bull. WHO. *31:*699, 1964.
6. Chin, W., Contacos, P., Coatney, G.
and King, H. The evaluation of sulfonamides, alone or in combination with pyrimethamine, in the treatment of multi-resistant f a l c i p a r u m malaria. *Amer. J. Trop. Med. 15:*823, 1966.
7. Bartelloni, P., Sheehy, T. and Tigertt, W. Combined therapy for chloroquine-resistant *Plasmodium falciparum* infection. *J.A.M.A. 199:*173, 1967.
8. Harinasuta, T., Viravan, C. and Reid, H. Sulphormethoxine in chloroquine-resistant falciparum malaria in Thailand. *Lancet. 1:*1117, 1967.
9. Laing, A. Treatment of acute falciparum malaria with diaphenylsulfone in North-East Tanzania. *J. Trop. Med. Hyg. 68:*251, 1965.
10. Degowin, R., Eppes, R., Carson, P. and Powell, R. The effects of diaphenylsulfone (DDS) against chloroquine-resistant *Plasmodium falciparum.* Bull. WHO. *34:*671, 1966.

11. Sheehy, T., Reba, R., Neff, T., Gaintner, J. and Tigertt, W. Supplemental sulfone (Dapsone) therapy. Use in treatment of chloroquine-resistant falciparum malaria. *Arch. Intern. Med. 119:*561, 1967.

12. Blount, R. Management of chloroquine-resistant falciparum malaria. *Arch. Intern. Med. 119:*557, 1967.

13. Gilbert, D., Moore, Jr., W., Hedberg, C. and Sanford, J. Potential medical problems in personnel returning from Vietnam. *Ann. Intern. Med. 68:*662, 1968.

14. Legters, L., Wallace D., Powell, R. and Pollack, S. Apparent refractoriness to chloroquine, pyrimethamine, and quinine in strains of *Plasmodium falciparum* from Vietnam. *Milit. Med. 130:* 168, 1965.

15. Blount, R. Acute falciparum malaria: Field experience with quinine/pyrimethamine combined therapy. *Ann. Intern. Med. 70:*142, 1969.

16. Martin, D. and Arnold, J. Treatment of acute falciparum malaria with sulfalene and trimethoprim. *J.A.M.A. 203:* 476, 1968.

17. Chin, W. and Contacos, P. G. Unpublished data.

# SYMPOSIUM ON MALARIA *

### General Discussion

Edited by

### KEVIN M. CAHILL

Director, The Tropical Disease Center
Associate Professor of Clinical Medicine
New York Medical College
New York, N. Y.

## Panelists

Harry Most, *chairman*          John Arnold
Brian Maegraith                 Peter G. Contacos

KEVIN M. CAHILL. This panel discussion provides an opportunity not only for its chairman, Harry Most, to elicit further details from our participants, but to give the audience an opportunity to ask questions.

DR. MOST. It is gratifying, after you have gone to the trouble to prepare a presentation, to have at least one person in the audience ask one question and so, before proceeding with the drug panel, we shall now invite questions. Are there any queries specifically directed to Irving G. Kagan, who gave a very illuminating and interesting presentation on the serologic diagnosis of malaria?

WALTER NAUENBERG. How long is the serologic reaction active?

DR. KAGAN. In order to answer this question, it is necessary to categorize the type of patient. If you are dealing with a susceptible person who has been in an endemic area for a short time and has come back with malaria (in this category is the Vietnam veteran who, incidentally, should he relapse with malaria in the United States, would receive curative treatment), the serologic reaction will become negative in approximately nine months. After six months, a titer of 1:256 by the fluorescent antibody method would indicate that the individual still has an active infection and should be treated again. In an endemic area, after malaria has been eradicated, we know that many individuals will have

---

*Held by The Tropical Disease Center, St. Clare's Hospital, New York, N. Y., and The Merck Company Foundation, Rahway, N. J., at the Center, May 17, 1969.

90

indirect hemagglutination titers for as long as five years and, according to a study made in Tobago, in the West Indies, about 10% for as long as 14 years. A titer may persist for many years at relatively high levels in an endemic area.

DR. MOST. Any other questions dealing with the serologic aspects?

LESLIE STAUBER. In the study of long-term malaria patients who were examined after 14 years, is there any information on possible anamnestic reactions? Did you ask the patients whether they had an acute febrile illness within, say, the last month? They might have an anamnestic response and this might be one kind of false-positive in those long-term cases.

DR. KAGAN. I think this is something that deserves continued study. We did not ask for any recent clinical history from these patients because malaria, as is well known, had been eradicated from Tobago for many years. It was of interest that the individuals in Tobago who were positive in 1969 were the oldest ones, in terms of age, in the group tested in 1955. I suspect that they had much more experience with malaria before the eradication period, which came into effect during the years 1953 to 1959. This finding suggests that for these people titers were dropping more slowly than the others tested in 1955.

DR. MOST. Are there any questions to address to George Fisher, who reviewed the problems of malaria in the United States, both imported and transfusion malaria, and other basic data.

BRIAN MAEGRAITH. One thing that interested me was the relatively small numbers of falciparum cases that were reported in people coming from overseas and also the small number of deaths. In the last two months in England, we have had several deaths from falciparum—five, I think—and this year I think we are going to have deaths from falciparum well into two figures. The total number of falciparum cases recorded in the last official figures, from 1967, was 92. Now to me that represents only a small proportion of the actual number of cases. In England, malaria is a reportable disease but I do not think that everybody reports it. In fact, in one *WHO Bulletin* I saw—I think it was in 1966—there had been six deaths in Britain and one case recorded, which takes quite a bit of biological understanding.

DR. MOST. Would you like to reply or comment, Dr. Fisher?

DR. FISHER. Let me comment first about the rarity of falciparum among returning troops. That is something that has struck us too, particularly since falciparum is far and away most common among the troops in Vietnam. I think there are probably several explanations. One is that a fair number of falciparum infections are probably resistant to chloroquine and therefore became manifest in Vietnam and are treated and cured there. Another is that the life-span of *P. falciparum* in the human host rarely exceeds one year, so many individuals who are infected early during their tour in Vietnam may naturally lose the parasite by the time they get back to the United States.

I share your feeling that notifiable diseases are not invariably reported but I think our malaria surveillance system is reasonably comprehensive and our data on malaria fatalities relatively accurate. I say this because in this country most of the malaria cases occur on the military bases and, the military situation being what it is, officials are required to report the cases: men are assigned to do this, and that is their job. I think we have an efficient surveillance system in the population and yet we do not observe as many fatalities as you cite. I think this is partly a reflection of the fact that military officials are keenly attuned to the possibility of the development of malaria in their troops and are quick to administer effective therapy.

One other remark I want to make is about some of the serologic data. Although the failure of an individual's antibody titer to fall below 256 six months after therapy might imply that that individual has not been cured, may I point out that if his titer has fallen to negative, it does not mean he is cured. We know that you cannot predict relapses with serologic techniques, probably because a parasitemia is necessary to boost the antibody response. Many men who returned from Vietnam have been treated for vivax malaria; their antibody titers had fallen to negative quickly and then subsequently they relapsed. So the present serologic tests are not effective in predicting who has lost the tissue stages and who has not.

Dr. Nauenberg. Are there any statistics on transfusion malaria in drug addicts?

Dr. Fisher. I know of no cases in the last three or four years that have been referred to the Communicable Disease Center in Atlanta. Ga. There was one possible case here in New York City but the drug addict had also received an exchange transfusion. We wondered, since the problem of drug use and the use of shared syringes probably has been on the increase, why there are not more cases than in the past. Howard

92

Shookoff of the Health Department here in New York City has suggested that the introduction of quinine as an adulterating agent into some of the heroin and other drugs that are used may be responsible for this.

DR. MOST. I do not believe that this is true. In the original epidemic, which Milton Helpern and I studied extensively in the 1930's, quinine and lactose were both used as adulterating agents. The risk of acquiring malaria became such common knowledge among drug addicts that any febrile disease they experienced stimulated them to treat themselves with adequate doses of quinine. In fact, I did a survey in the Tombs Prison among drug addicts with no history of illness and found gametocytes in their blood, which indicated that they had an infection and that they were taking quinine. I think that the main reason that drug addicts now do not have malaria is not that they are not exposed; the reason is a simple arithmetical one. I think that disposable syringes are so readily available that it is not necessary for them to use a spoon, an eye dropper, and a medicine bulb to take their heroin jointly. I think they take it independently and that they use disposable syringes freely.

DAVID GOLDSTEIN. I think that this is not quite true. I think addicts do exchange the syringe and needle, although they do not still use the eye dropper and the needle. They do not have enough syringes to go around and so there is common usage. We have been doing routine urines for narcotics on our preemployment examinations and, in the first 10 positive urines that we obtained, none of the patients were "mainliners," and some denied drug use or abuse. Incidentally, we found that half of the group had a history of infectious hepatitis. We obtained abstracts from the hospital and in each instance it was diagnosed as infectious hepatitis. It could have been infectious hepatitis, but this incidence is a very high one and, despite the fact that it is from a small sample, I suspect strongly that most of them had homologous serum jaundice. If they had, then in the case of our returning Vietnamese troops—many of whom are addicts, as we have found—we may still have a potential problem. Quinine is regularly used and appears regularly in the urine long after the drug disappears; it lasts for five to six days in the urine. On the West Coast lactose is the diluent, but on the East Coast quite uniformly quinine is used.

DR. MOST. I now ask you if you have any questions to address to Craig Canfield.

Dr. Fisher. I should appreciate hearing what Dr. Maegraith has to say about this, too. I was interested by a paper in the literature recently in which the use of heparin was investigated in simian malaria. The interest of the authors was stimulated by the description of consumptive coagulopathy in malaria and the possible therapeutic effect of heparin in individuals who develop this complication. Heparin was administered to a group of monkeys at the time they were infected; a control group was also infected but did not receive heparin. What they found, to their surprise, was that the heparin-treated monkeys never developed a parasitemia whereas the control group all developed a parasitemia and all died from their malaria. This would imply to me that heparin has an antimalarial action that is divorced from its action as an anticoagulant. I wonder if Dr. Canfield or anyone else has had an experience with heparin as an antimalarial or if they have any speculations about it.

Dr. Canfield. I should be interested in hearing Dr. Maegraith's comments on this also. A point that I should like to make about the use of heparin in patients with evidence of consumptive coagulopathy in acute malaria infections is that it needs further study. I am not sure we are at a point where we should start treating all patients with acute falciparum malaria with heparin, even with evidence of consumptive coagulopathy, primarily because the patients, as I have indicated in my paper, that have been treated this way have also received antimalarial medications so that we cannot separate one from another. More work does need to be done in animal models to try and delineate the difference between the heparin activity and the antimalarial activity.

Dr. Maegraith. I am under the impression that when the heparin was stopped the parasites came back and, if that is the case, then I think this is a blocking, rather similar to the effect you get when you put an animal on milk—the parasite disappears. So far as using anticoagulants is concerned, we are now using arvin. Arvin is an extract from the venom of the pit viper (*Agkistrodon*) and has the peculiarity amongst all anticoagulant agents that it is a defibrinator and nothing else. I think possibly this might lead to better information.

Dr. Most. I can add to Dr. Maegraith's statement regarding the use of heparin in severe *P. knowlesi* infections in monkeys. When the heparin is discontinued, all the monkeys become infected and die, so it has only a temporary suppressive effect. As I indicated to Dr. Canfield before, this is a laboratory observation. If you recall the lesions I showed in the brain and in the vessels where there is already bleeding and transudation of red cells through capillaries that are permeable, you would be reluctant to try to overcome a laboratory coagulation defect clinically because of the danger of having major additional hemorrhage and extensive damage in the brain.

Let us now go on to the formal aspects of the panel's function, namely a discussion of the chemotherapy of malaria. I have a series of questions first that I shall put to the speakers, and then perhaps the audience can build on these comments for additional questions.

In the drugs that have been presented, both old and new, very little was brought out with regard to side effects and toxicity of the drugs now employed, whether from single or prolonged use. I address these remarks to John Arnold for his comments.

DR. ARNOLD. First, the design of an antimalarial drug is like almost no other pharmaceutical enterprise. The requirements concerning adverse effects and ease of administration seem almost insurmountable. The drugs are used by lay people who have not even the ability to read and write, and they are administered on a broad scale even in the absence of malaria. They are given to anybody, and medical supervision is rare. So we have a double standard here, for side effects or adverse effects in an antimalarial can be much more important than they would be, let us say, in an important antibacterial compound used in the United States. I think—and these opinions are my own—that all antimalarial drugs should have one adverse effect. That one adverse effect ought to be nausea and vomiting when the dose is too large and, if this effect is not in the drug as it comes from the chemist, I think maybe it ought to be put there. This effect from overdosage would prevent some really unfortunate things that have resulted from the use of antimalarials under field conditions.

In describing the adverse effects of the drugs now used, let us start with chloroquine. At the dose that chloroquine should be used it is a remarkable drug. It is now a favorite custom to declaim about chloroquine resistance, chloroquine retinopathy, and other such factors, but this drug has been used for 20 years, and it is still considered a remarkable drug. I do not think we shall ever find one better. The adverse effects of chloroquine for the most part may be due to overdosage.

Primaquine, I think, is another matter. Primaquine, as I have indicated earlier, has barely sufficed. It has never been as satisfactory a drug as chloroquine, and it must be given in much narrower tolerances. It bothers many persons, and gastrointestinal distress often results at the required doses. Of course, you say, that is what is wanted in the drug, and that is correct, but I should like to have it at a little higher dosage and have fewer people complain about it. There is a percentage, 10 or 20%, of persons on the present CP (chloroquine-primaquine) program who have gastrointestinal distress. I have gastrointestinal distress. Primaquine also causes hemolysis but, in the vast majority of cases, this is a self-limited problem. I think Dr. Canfield may know more about this than I do, but the number of serious accidents in the military service from primaquine hemolysis is almost negligible. This is surprising, as 10% of American Negroes have primaquine-sensitive erythrocytes, but there is a sort of control mechanism here that keeps this from amounting to anything. I am not aware of any significant incidence of agranulocytosis from this drug either; so, by and large, results have been fairly satisfactory.

DR. MOST. I think, then, one can consider these findings very reassuring, particularly in regard to what was available before, namely, atabrine. We are not faced with extensive numbers of individuals with exfoliative dermatitis, aplastic anemia, atypical lichen planus, and other complicating, serious, disabling, and associated fatal reactions. I reiterate this because not infrequently the questions of the toxicity and the tolerability of the drugs now available are overemphasized, and I think we must face the reality that these are the best drugs and the only ones to use.

There is a very expensive military program for finding new agents that will be better than chloroquine as a suppressive and therapeutic agent, that will overcome the problem of resistance, and that will be superior to primaquine as a definitively curative drug. Peter G. Contacos: can you comment on the present status of any promising new agents?

DR. CONTACOS. In this regard, as you just stated, the U. S. Army has a very large program in operation. My personal experience and the experience of our group at the National Institutes of Health (NIH) has been with several compounds, the foremost of which is known as RC-12, a pyrocatechol. Leon Schmidt, formerly at the Primate Center in Palto Alto, Calif., and, in fact, our group also, have studied the effectiveness of this compound against simian malaria, and all indications are that it has excellent prophylactic activity. When this drug was administered to monkeys by the fourth day after exposure and continued for five consecutive days (the dosage was roughly 25 mg./kg. body weight), complete protection was obtained. In fact, some recent studies have indicated that treating monkeys once a week with the same dose and exposing them repeatedly to simian malaria protected all the animals so treated. When we finally took the animals off medication they were observed for four to eight weeks. Then we splenectomized them and followed them for an additional four weeks. Almost invariably after splenectomy in monkeys, if there are residual tissue stages, latent infection will become evident. Every one of these animals remained negative. Unfortunately the ratio between therapeutic effect and toxicity observed in the monkeys was not great enough, and there has been a reluctance to allow us to use this compound on inmate volunteers. This is where we stand at the moment with this compound. There are some analogs of lincomycin that have been studied by one of my colleagues at NIH and also by Dr. Schmidt. One of these analogs has also apparently shown some excellent activity. We hope that possibly some day we can try this on volunteers.

Dr. Most. Dr. Arnold mentioned that sulfones, or one form of sulfone, had promise in terms of being administered weekly, together with chloroquine and primaquine, instead of daily.

What this will amount to, then, is that the suppressive schedule overseas will consist of 500 mg. of chloroquine salt, 45 mg. of primaquine salt, and 800 to 1600 mg. of a long-acting diformol-diaminodiphenyl sulfone (DDS).

The only things new on the horizon that have not gone beyond the stage of study by the Food and Drug Administration are drugs from World War II, which were very effective in trials but which had the alarming property of phototoxicity. These compounds have been modified in such a way that their potential toxicity has been removed, but pharmacological and clinical applications of these drugs will not be feasible for some time.

Dr. Maegraith. Can you report for the Commonwealth and for Great Britain any great promise of new agents?

Dr. Maegraith. The simple answer is: "No." I do not think there are any at the moment, but could I come back to Dr. Arnold on a point? I was a little disappointed, as a member of the original team which produced paludrine, to hear so little about proguanil in your conversations. I wondered why. I believe you have tried it extensively. It is being extensively used in the Australian Army with reasonably good results. Sometimes in periods of high transmission it may be topped with DDS to catch the odd paludrine-resistant strain. I should like to know whether these resistant strains that the troops are getting are being transmitted to them from one to another via mosquito or whether you think they derive from the local population.

DR. ARNOLD. The present evidence is that they come from the local population. I have been told that the intelligence officers in Vietnam usually suspect the infiltration of North Vietnamese when there is a rising incidence of malaria in the troops in a given region; the chloroquine resistance to this malaria is a tip-off as to its origin. There is much evidence that this originates along the Ho Chi Minh trail in Laos and Cambodia, and in the western highlands. It is carried largely by the North Vietnamese, who are now carrying incidences of this kind of malaria up to 50% to 100%.

DR. MOST. I think this is a rational explanation on several theoretical grounds, one of which is that in nonimmune groups such as American military personnel, drugs such as chloroquine, with a very great gap between the suppressive level and the achieved plasma concentration, will eradicate most of the parasites and transmission. However, in immune individuals who tolerate parasitemia without symptoms or disease, the mutation or the basis for the generation of mutant resistant strains is greater and therefore the transmission among them is greater, as is their transmission to us.

DR. MAEGRAITH. You did not say why you are not using proguanil.

DR. MOST. I can give you one reason: It must be given every day. Another reason is that the speed of action in falciparum disease is significantly less than that of chloroquine or quinine, and if there is failure or faulty suppressive discipline in taking the drug, and if disease occurs and you are relying on this drug, then the probability of having a suitable outcome in severe falciparum disease is compromised.

DR. MAEGRAITH. I do not think much of your first answer. Proguanil works in Australians and I think if any treatment works in Australians, it should work quite easily in Americans. A second point that I think you are missing is the fact that proguanil acts on the preerythrocytic cycle, so it should act before other drugs do.

98

Dr. Most. We have taken much criticism about this—the Australians have been pushing us pretty hard about it—because the Australian Army did have a fine record until recently, but now we are on even terms with them. Apparently this was partly a result of the localities in which the Australians were stationed. The Australians were on the sea coast, which was apparently not a very endemic area, and the recent movement of an Australian group to the Central Highlands resulted in a high rate of malaria. All these arguments, of course, are meaningless if proguanil works.

Dr. Maegraith. I cannot answer you because the information is classified. I am not trying to avoid the point, but I think this is probably not correct. The second thing is that it is fairly easy to produce paludrine resistance on therapeutic dosage but not so easy to produce it on the ordinary level of suppression, so I think you ought to give it a trial.

Dr. Arnold. One other thing is that cross-resistance with pyrimethamine is almost complete and that most of these strains are pyrimethamine resistant.

Dr. Most. The management of the complications which have been presented by the speakers, I think, are self-evident in terms of the pathophysiology, and I do not think the panel needs to go into this. I had it listed as one of the possible bases for interpanel discussion but if members of the audience are interested, I think we are in a position to discuss the management of the pathophysiological changes which have been presented: namely, the renal insufficiency, the coagulation defect, the cardiovascular changes, the shock syndrome, and the anoxemic situation with regard to anemia. Comment has not been made on hyperbilirubinemia and on the predominant cerebral manifestations.

Does any member of the panel wish to say anything about the possible role of genetic defects of the host in relation to its response in malaria? We have already had comment on the deficiency of the given enzyme which might enhance the toxicity or tolerability of aminoquinolines. Are there any others that any of you know?

Dr. Maegraith. I know of no others, but a little experimental work has recently been done by Kanika in Bangkok in which she has measured the production of free hemoglobin in the plasma during induced falciparum malaria. She chose equal numbers of persons deficient in glucose-6-phosphate dehydrogenase and normal people, and she found no appreciable difference between the members of these two groups.

DR. Most. I should now like to open the discussion to questions from the audience.

KEVIN M. CAHILL. Dr. Maegraith implied that he did not see a great role for the use of steroids earlier in the discussion. Could you or Dr. Contacos comment on indications for the use of steroids in cerebral malaria?

DR. Most. Dr. Maegraith provides great reliance on the efficacy of quinine and chloroquine in stopping this free transport of protein and perhaps the fluid of vessels and of endothelial capillary vessels and the surrounding tissue. My feeling perhaps is one of alarm, at least in regard to a patient in coma who is already compromised with a high degree of parasitemia: particularly, as Dr. Fisher pointed out, when there is this lag in days between onset and diagnosis and perhaps irreversible damage. Perhaps this is empiricism on my part, but I should feel the legal and the moral pressure to give steroids on the basis that these perhaps are the most effective agents in reducing cerebral edema.

DR. CAHILL. I agree with that approach.

DR. GOLDSTEIN. I am still a little confused about suppressive therapy. The problem is a very common one, much more so than treatment of disease, I hasten to mention. Family physicians call me frequently about employees in various industries as to what program of immunization should be given and, in addition, whether malarial prophylaxis is indicated. I have become somewhat better informed today in regard to some of those areas where malaria has been eliminated and where it has broken out again, as in Ceylon and South America, but I am not sure about this area. We have been told that where there is no chloroquine-resistant falciparum, chloroquine alone is adequate for suppressive therapy. What is the exact dosage of antimalarial advised as a prophylaxis for those about to visit nonchloroquine-resistant areas?

DR. Most. Two tablets of aralen (250 mg.) once weekly. Dr. Maegraith, do you want to make a recommendation on the routine chemosuppression?

DR. MAEGRAITH. I advise my patients to take proguanil. I do this because I think it is a general-usage drug that is easy to take. Persons in private life, at any rate, can quite often manage a drug once a day better than they can once a week. I think it is different when they are under discipline. And there are persons who spend most of their time in tropical cities such as Bangkok, where air conditioning abounds, who are suddenly called to the bush, say just for a few days. I think such persons should be regarded as fully exposed to malaria and that they must be subjected to a full regime. One of the fatal cases we had recently was in a man on a cruise whose ship stopped at Lagos. He was in Lagos for only six hours and this was the only endemic area visited on the trip. I know of a woman who died in South Africa from missed falciparum malaria whose only exposure was the stop-off at Kano, Nigeria, while the plane refueled. It takes one mosquito half a minute to infect anyone. If one is going to suppress, then one should suppress fully.

Dr. FISHER. I should like to ask if you would be willing to commit yourselves as to chemoprophylaxis administered during pregnancy. This problem comes to our attention very frequently also. For instance, the Peace Corps is willing to transport pregnant Peace Corps volunteers out of the malarious area rather than administer chloroquine during the first trimester. There is a report in the literature of vestibular abnormalities in two children of a mother who was taking chloroquine in dosages much greater than those used for suppression. She had systemic lupus, I believe. But this problem comes to our attention frequently, and I think most physicians, rightly so, are very reluctant to administer any drugs that are not absolutely needed in the first trimester of pregnancy. We have frequently just thrown up our hands and have said it is a difficult question to answer. I wonder if you are willing to commit yourselves on this point.

JOHN FRAME. I take care of Protestant missionaries and their families. During the past 15 years I have taken care of approximately 1,000 women of the child-bearing age who have taken chloroquine for varying periods. I do not know of a single complication from this drug, and I have very good records on these women and their children. There are about 3,500 children in these families. I do not know of any case of teratogenecity we could ascribe to chloroquine. I do know of two or three persons who had children born with major deformities, but these have been divided between those who have taken chloroquine and those who never did. I think statistically we could say that chloroquine probably can be completely acquitted of responsibility. I just do not feel there is any danger, though I should like to study my own material statistically one of these days.

DR. GOLDSTEIN. The wife of one of our correspondents who is going to India and to such areas as Celyon wants to go with him on his travels and she wants to become pregnant. The question she asked me on Friday (when I said I was coming before the world's leading experts and should certainly have an answer for her on Monday) is, "Are there any teratogenetic effects from sustained prophylactic therapy or actual treatment of the acute disease?" Is there any knowledge of this?

DR. CAHILL. There are no such reports. Chloroquine has been very widely used for many years throughout the world and there are no documented examples of human teratogenic side effects. Further extensive animal studies with chloroquine have also failed to produce any fetal changes attributable to the drug. Chloroquine, therefore, can be prescribed for women at all stages of pregnancy, and should be prescribed for those entering malarious areas.

DR. ARNOLD. One thing we can say for sure is that none of these antimalarials will help your patient become pregnant.

DR. MAEGRAITH. One experiment we did accidentally during the war may encourage Dr. Goldstein. When I was directing research for the British Army on mepacrine, my group comprised 50 people. In two years these persons produced 11 healthy children.

DR. MOST. This, incidentally, was to counteract word-of-mouth rumors to troops that they should not take atabrine because it not only made one yellow but also sterile.

Perhaps Dr. Goldstein's problem is unique in the sense that correspondents may go into war zones. But, as has been said, when one is in cities where air conditioning exists, particularly in areas where there is no problem of chloroquine resistance, then chloroquine is the drug usually prescribed in the United States for travelers leaving the country. With regard to the use of primaquine after exposure, I think it is incumbent on the physician to have some knowledge of what the relapse potential is and how serious the exposure has been. Strains originating from the Mediterranean have a relapse potential of only about 30% compared to those originating in New Guinea, which have a relapse potential after chloroquine, paludrine, or quinine, or anything else, of 90%. One must define not only the arithmetic probability but the geographic origin of the strain, and then one can decide about giving primaquine for 14 days.

DR. CAHILL. Would one of the panelists comment on the age at which antimalarial prophylaxis should be started in an infant born or going to be born in a malarious area? What is the best prophylactic drug to use in a pediatric group and what are the optimal dosages?

DR. MOST. I recommend chloroquine. Those under 15 lb. should receive 62.5 mg. weekly; those from 15 to 30 lb. should receive 125 mg.; those from 30 to 60 lb. should receive 250 mg.; and those over 60 lb. should be given a full adult dose of 500 mg. aralen (300 mg. chloroquine base). Adults and children should begin prophylaxis when they enter the malarious area.

DR. GOLDSTEIN. How long after the removal of a person from a malarious area do you continue the use of chloroquine for suppressive treatment?

DR MOST. The usual period is four weeks from the last possible exposure.

JAMIL HADDAD. I wonder if this distinguished panel could give us a guide as to the acceptability of persons who have contracted malaria as future blood donors. How many years later could we use them for blood donation? As far as I know, up till now, the laws state that such persons may donate.

DR. MOST. This has been a moot question. Dr. Fischer has commented on the removal of those who have had malaria. In fact, you know, perhaps, as director of the blood bank in this hospital, that there are guide lines with regard to the use of donors in relation to malaria. The armed forces' Epidemiology Board's commission on malaria did not see fit to change these guide lines for a number of reasons. Perhaps, Dr. Fisher, you would like to reiterate what you said and emphasize the present basic rules of blood banks and of the American Red Cross.

DR. FISHER. The screening criteria are based on life-span of the parasite in the human host, which varies with the species. *Plasmodium malariae* may persist for up to 40 years, *P. falciparum* is generally thought not to persist more than a year or so, and *P. vivax* may persist for two or three years. Most blood banks reject anyone who has a history of malaria or a history of travel to malarious areas within two years of their attacks or after their return from such areas. We know from our experience that application of such criteria would exclude a fair number of the cases that have occurred, but it would fail to exclude some of the *Plasmodium malariae* infections and also would fail, it seems, to exclude some of the falciparum infections. As I have pointed out, it has been our experience in this country that most of the *Plasmodium malariae* donors are foreign immigrants or visitors from foreign countries. Whether exclusion of all such individuals would reduce significantly the incidence of quartan malaria after transfusions would have to be seen. We shall not know until such an experiment has been tried. There is the added problem that such persons may comprise a significant segment of the current donor pool, and I do not have any data on that subject either. These criteria are nice to have, but whether they are applied by most blood banks is another question. If more strict application of current criteria were applied, we might have fewer cases.

DR. MOST. Let us consider an emergency in which one must use blood and the donor does not come from an area where there is chloroquine resistance (in which case one would exclude the donor). Even if the donor has a history of malaria, but comes from an area where there is no known resistance, I believe that one could safely use that blood in an emergency and, simultaneously or soon thereafter, give the recipient about a gram of chloroquine to wipe out the asexual parasites, which then would not become established and produce a subsequent relapse. Now this might have legal disadvantages, but I think that in an emergency I should not hesitate to do that.

LEONARD SCHIEBEL. Dr. Maegraith's comment on the good fortune of the Australian boys who took proguanil reminds me that about a year ago General William D. Tigertt, who was heading a program in a symposium at Johns Hopkins, pointed out that the Australian and the New Zealand boys did have the good fortune of not coming down with as much malaria as the American troops. When the sun went down the Australians' sleeves went down, their head nettings went on, they slept under mosquito netting at night, and they used mosquito repellent. It was 18 to 21 months ago that he made that comment. The Americans were not so scrupulous at that time, and he felt that this was the reason.

DR. MAEGRAITH. As an Australian, I do not think there is any need for comment.

DR. MOST. Before we close, I should like to take the liberty of inviting Victor G. Heiser, who at the age of 97 is our senior tropical-disease man here, to offer some comments relative to this symposium.

DR. HEISER. What happened long ago may not be of much interest now, but I am reminded of a story about two hippies. You may have heard it. Two hippies, walking down a street, encountered a Catholic priest who was limping along on a crutch, and they asked him what happened; the priest said he fell in the bath and broke his leg. After he got out of earshot one hippie said to the other, "What's a bath?" The other fellow replied: "How should I know? I'm not a Catholic."

So much of the discussion has been on quinine today. Many of you here are probably not too familiar with things that happened during World War I. The Dutch raised the price of quinine to fantastic heights and, at the end of the war, the British, determined to break that monopoly, asked the Dutch to supply them with some slips which they planted in the hills in the Madras Residency. When the trees began to bear, the Dutch came in and sold quinine cheaper than the British could take it from their own trees. That made the British angry, and they managed to get a secret-service man on the job. The Dutch monopoly in Java was fenced in completely; there were guards day and night to see that nobody got into the area where the Dutch had their cinchona trees. But the British managed to get in an agent who found that the Dutch had given the British slips from trees that had been abandoned. Meanwhile the Dutch had developed trees that produced five times as much cinchona as the ones they gave to the British.

# SYMPOSIUM ON AMEBIASIS

## Introduction*

### KEVIN M. CAHILL, M.D.

Director
Tropical Disease Center
St. Clare's Hospital and Health Center
New York, N. Y.
Professor of Tropical Medicine
Royal College of Surgeons
Dublin, Ireland

A MEBIASIS holds an interesting position in the constellation of "tropical" diseases in temperate climates. In North America we have experienced some of the greatest water-borne epidemics of invasive amebiasis known to man, most notably the Chicago epidemic in 1933 and the outbreak in South Bend, Ind., in 1956. Numerous stool surveys among random populations have shown an incidence ranging from 1% to more than 10%, the vast majority of subjects being asymptomatic. During the first part of this century the causative parasite, *Entamoeba histolytica*, was regarded by most physicians as universally harmful to man. In recent years the pendulum of opinion as to pathogenicity has swung so far that some consider intestinal cysts of *E. histolytica* to be merely commensal protozoa.

---

*Presented as part of a *Symposium on Amebiasis* sponsored by The Tropical Disease Center, St. Clare's Hospital, New York, N. Y., and The Merck Company Foundation, Rahway, N. J., held at the Center, September 12, 1970.

Amebiasis is often, usually unfairly, regarded as the bête noire of the traveler, and is probably the most often misdiagnosed ailment of American tourists. Recognition of the etiologic organism requires appropriate laboratory techniques and—equally important—an adequately trained parasitology technician; both are frequently wanting in general hospitals. However, one has to work as a clinician for only a brief period in any of the developing lands to appreciate what great problems amebic dysentery and intestinal amebiasis are, and one has to observe but a few patients devastated by amebiasis to recognize its full potency. It will be noted later in this symposium that amebiasis is the most common cause of admission to some hospitals in Africa, and the most common cause of death. Tragically—since the correct diagnosis can almost always be made *if* an awareness of the possibility exists, and treatment is almost always fully effective *if* it is provided early enough—deaths also still occur in New York City from amebiasis.

It is obviously crucial to define amebiasis. What are the criteria for labeling one protozoon, *E. histolytica*, as pathogenic and relieving another of this opprobrium? Are there different strains of *E. histolytica?* What does the organism do in the human body? Can we correlate *in vitro* experiments with our clinical experience? None of these questions is easy to answer and yet a start must be made. As with previous symposia on clinical tropical medicine published in the *Bulletin of the New York Academy of Medicine*, our attempt has been to provide a comprehensive view of an important clinical topic.

We begin with the epidemiology of amebiasis around the world, as viewed by Dr. Ronald Elsdon-Dew, director of the Amebiasis Research Institute in Durban, South Africa, and by Dr. Kerrison Juniper, Jr., of Arkansas, in the United States. Dr. R. A. Neal's studies on the organism itself provide the link between the epidemiologic studies and offer a basis for our consideration of the clinical picture. Few physicians have had the opportunity of working at a hospital that admits 5,000 cases of proved amebiasis per year. This vast experience with clinical patterns of and therapeutic approaches to clinical amebiasis is summarized by Dr. S. John Powell. The difficulties of diagnosing amebiasis, especially in smaller hospitals where experienced parasitological technicians are rare, is considered by the head of the Protozoology Section at our National Center for Communicable Diseases in Atlanta, Ga. Dr. Healy's emphasis on classic parasitologic techniques provides an introduction to the newest and crucial phase in our understanding of "invasive" as opposed to "commensal" amebiasis. During the last 10 years various laboratory techniques have been employed to detect the presence of circulating antibody against *E. histolytica*. These have proved valuable as seroepidemiologic tools and as aids to the clinican who deals with extraintestinal amebiasis and, to a lesser degree, with intestinal infection.

In summary, this is another in a series of symposia the goal of which is to provide the clinician in the developed world with improved knowledge of the "tropical" diseases that are appearing in ever increasing numbers in this country as Americans travel, as soldiers return, and as the good physician's diagnostic index of suspicion rises.

# AMEBIASIS AS A WORLD PROBLEM*

RONALD ELSDON-DEW, M.D.

Director
Amebiasis Research Unit
Durban, South Africa

IT might seem strange that one who has worked with this disease for
25 years and more should now be acting as counsel for the defense
for *Entamoeba histolytica*. Perhaps it was because one was confronted
with the flagrant manifestations as seen in our Bantu peoples that one
realized just what the parasite could do, and yet there were people
harboring the parasite in whom the clinical manifestations were so
vague as to defy classification.

I have been called an iconoclast and an agent provocateur, but
I have followed the advice given many years ago of an older scientist
who said to me: "Young man, if you want to get on in science—establish a heresy!"

But let us go back into ancient history and see how the many
misconceptions about *Entamoeba histolytica* arose. The early observers
were indeed astute. Long before the discovery of the ameba by Friedrich
Lösch in 1875, physicians practicing in India were well aware of more
than one kind of dysentery; some of the cases were followed by hepatic
abscess. Ballingall[1] refers to "acute colonitis" and the "hepatic flux."
He pointed out that the dependent portions of the colon were particularly affected by the latter. He relates the story of "an officer of the
Madras establishment having had an abscess of the liver opened by his
adversary's ball, in fighting a duel, and by this means obtaining a complete cure." He himself used "the introduction of a seton" as a means
of treating such abscesses.

I have repeatedly recommended perusal of the original description
of the ameba and its manifestations by Lösch.[2] When one considers the
available equipment, this article is a model of investigative technique
and deduction. Though this article is much quoted, it is only too appar-

*Presented as part of a *Symposium on Amebiasis* sponsored by The Tropical Disease Center, St. Clare's Hospital. New York, N. Y., and The Merck Company Foundation, Rahway, N.J., held at the Center, September 12, 1970.

ent from statements made that but few of the writers had consulted the original masterpiece.

Such casuistry is well illustrated by the many references to "O.Uplavici," which means "on dysentery" in Bohemian; the other authority was Hlava.[3] This however was a fault of the 20th century; the 19th century observers were much more honest.

Perhaps the best description of the clinical presentation and pathology came from Johns Hopkins University in Baltimore in 1891 by Councilman and Lafleur.[4] Here too is a classic which all interested persons should read. Characteristic is the comment that what is called an amebic abscess in the liver is not inflammatory but "caused by necrosis, softening and liquefaction of the tissue." The authors also stated that in the liver the amebas were not associated with other organisms.

Though Casagrandi and Barbagallo[5] had described *Entamoeba coli* from healthy persons, it was Schaudinn[6] who, in 1903, distinguished between this and the hematophagous ameba *Entamoeba histolytica* which now bears his name. However he can be regarded as having started the confusion which was to bedevil our ideas on amebiasis for so many years. It was of course Schaudinn who, by describing the direct entry of the malarial sporozoite into a red blood cell, similarly retarded our recognition of the exoerythrocytic phase of malaria.

Schaudinn described the reproduction of *E. histolytica* by the budding off of nuclear chromatin. According to him these small buds formed resistant capsules that became spores which were resistant to complete drying. He also described schizogony in *E. coli*. Dobell[7] described these observations as "so incredible that it is difficult to believe that they were not sheer inventions."

But who could question the "Herr Professor"? When Hüber[8] demonstrated quadrinucleate cysts, his master, Schaudinn, told him that these belonged to another species which he proposed to call *"Entamoeba tetragena."* This belief remained unquestioned for many years, and attempts were made to rationalize the concept. Some investigators, including Hartmann[9] and Hüber,[10] accepted *E. tetragena* as a separate species. Viereck[11] considered it a variant of *E. coli*, and Elmassian[12] gave the name *Entamoeba minuta* to the nonhematophagous trophozoites he found associated with quadrinucleate cysts.

It is perhaps a sorry fact that the papers of Walker[13, 14] and of

Walker and Sellards[15] appeared in such obscure journals, for they cannot have been read as widely as they have been quoted. Walker first showed that the names *tetragena* and *minuta* applied to phases of *E. histolytica* and thereafter he and his colleague Sellards carried out their famous experiment which showed the difference in pathogenicity between *E. histolytica* and *E. coli*. There is far more to this experiment than is generally appreciated. In addition to showing that *E. coli* did not give rise to dysentery, it also showed that *E. histolytica* did not always cause disease. A glance at a strain flow sheet based on their findings reveals that of 18 successful infections only four developed dysentery with hematophagous trophozoites. It is noteworthy that none of the dysenteric cases had been infected from active cases though the latter were able to colonize new cases. Walker and Sellards comment on this "latency"; they postulated that the amebas might be thought of as commensals.

In the same year (1913) Kuenen and Swellengrebel[16] postulated that there were three phases: an invasive *histolytica* phase, a commensal *minuta* phase, and the cystic *tetragena* phase necessary for transmission. Where Walker and Sellards had regarded the *minuta* phase as precystic and intervening between the *histolytica* and the cystic phases, Kuenen and Swellengrebel had considered the *histolytica* phase as a 'metamorphosis' of the commensal *minuta* phase.

Mathis and Mercier[17] pointed out that, as the *histolytica* phase is to be found only in the mucosanguineous stools of dysenteric patients, it could play no part in the evolutionary cycle of the parasite. The cycle was maintained by the *minuta* and cystic phases.

Thus the concept of the normal commensalism of *E. histolytica* had been promulgated more than 50 years ago, but the idea was vociferously attacked by authoritative workers, notably Dobell,[7, 18] who insisted that *E. histolytica* "lives in and on the living tissues of its host, and it can exist in no other way." Dobell thus established the Promethean school, which was to give rise to so much unnecessary treatment and hardship when it was championed by such American writers as Craig and Faust,[19] D'Antoni,[20] and others.

Once it was appreciated that the *tetragena* cysts were those of *E. histolytica* the worldwide distribution of the parasite was established and it was found in many persons who did not show any such classical signs as dysentery and liver abscess. But the Promethean school soon found a pathology, real or imaginary, to associate with the parasite. The list of conditions attributed to *E. histolytica* would fill a textbook and more, and it is unnecessary to enumerate them.

Perhaps my own early experience with the disease is illustrative of the danger of blindly adhering to the dicta of the pundits. When I first came to Durban, South Africa, the "ameba" was on everybody's lips, if not in their bowels. The hospitals and nursing homes all had a full quota of patients undergoing what could be called only vicious treatment. Emetine was the order of the day, with much obscenity in the form of bowel washouts and the like. My first study covered two hospitals, one for the white population and the other for the Bantu. It was not long before I appreciated the apparent difference between the two. In the Bantu the common presentations were classical dysentery or liver abscess, whereas those white patients diagnosed as having amebiasis usually showed vague symptoms often unrelated to the bowel. At that time I accepted, on the one hand, the clinical labeling and, on the other, the concepts of my Promethean teachers; I accordingly thought that the parasite affected the two races in different ways.

I made my unsuccessful attempts to elucidate this difference, but increasing experience, not only in Durban but in other parts of the world, led me to appreciate that the symptomatology in white patients had nothing to do with the ameba. In many parts of the world the ameba was being used as a scapegoat for the physicians' inability to make a diagnosis. Amebiasis was the regular resort of the diagnostically destitute. Unscrupulous physicians found the diagnosis lucrative, and in one American city I visited I was driven to say "Amebiasis is apparently a disease of those who can afford it."

Had I read the work of Reichenow[21, 22] earlier, I should have realized that, were they all feeding on the mucosa, the progenitors of the enormous number of cysts passed by a "carrier" could not but have given rise to colitis and dysentery.

Hoare[23, 24] deserves credit for the final condemnation of the Promethean concept, but his publications appeared in specialty journals and did not reach the physicians who were most concerned.

I now think the commensalist concept of Swellengrebel has reached almost complete acceptance except possibly by those who have a vested interest in maintaining the bad old days. When I[25] suggested the term lumenal amebiasis as a contrast to invasive amebiasis I was shouted down. My learned listeners approved the term asymptomatic amebiasis but could not countenance the possibility of a harmless *Entamoeba histolytica*. Now, I hope, this essential distinction between infection and disease is acceptable.

There were other confusing issues. It took a long time for the work of Sapero, Hankansson, and Louttit[26] to be appreciated. The spate of species-splitting which occurred in the second decade of this century made people reluctant to accept *Entamoeba hartmanni* as a species which might be mistaken for *E. histolytica*, and many a battle was fought. Recently, of course, "Laredo" has provided a further issue; it reminds us that morphology alone may mislead the experts. Then just how dangerous it is to leave fecal protozoology to the mercies of inadequately trained technicians. Many "epidemics" have followed the arrival of some new laboratorian!

Except where there is hematophagy, the finding of *E. histolytica sensustricto* in a patient's stool tells us but little. But had the old fashioned idea that hematophagy was the only criterion been adhered to, much unnesessary treatment and no little suffering would have been avoided.

However the disease is very real, for when *Entamoeba histolytica* invades the tissues it does considerable damage, as we in Durban know only too well. Perhaps in one way we have been fortunate in that the plethora of genuine cases has allowed us not only to make the contrast, but also to assess other factors. We have been able to evaluate treatment on the basis of strict criteria seldom attainable elsewhere. This is not the place to tell of the tribulations of testing one drug after another. Suffice it to say that metronidazole has completely changed the picture of treatment.

The other advantage we have had is the close association between the laboratory and the wards. This has meant that not only were our cases adequately documented, but queried points could be reexamined and discussed. It was this adequate documentation which has allowed us to put serology on a working basis. It is no use trying to evaluate a test without completely definitive test material. As we are to talk later on serology, I shall say no more at this stage.

I have made several attempts to evaluate the world situation in amebiasis. Perhaps the most heartening of these was a review carried out at the instigation of the World Health Organization (Elsdon-

114

Dew[27]). In this I evaluated the literature on the incidence of the parasite; ultimately I selected about 700 references. The chaos was such that my final comment was: "The only value of this report is to show that it has none!"

Though fecal protozoology is perhaps the most difficult of all routine laboratory procedures, it is regularly left to inadequately trained personnel, whose not-so-inspired guesses may set in train a long and uncomfortable period for the patient. What I have termed the pepper-pot technician is by no means uncommon. To justify his existence he must periodically find some pathogen, and he usually distributes these "positive" findings with fine abandon. The uninhibited enthusiasm of the uninitiated is to be matched only by the careful caution of the expert.

But even experts may be misled. Just how long did it take *Entamoeba hartmanni* to be recognized? The least said about Laredo the better, but this should convince most of the danger of depending on morphology alone. Small wonder that I could make no sense out of the world statistics.

I tried other approaches. The protean symptoms attributed to the ameba by the Promethean school made a direct analysis of clinical reports impossible. *Entamoeba histolytica* has been blamed for practically every clinical syndrome—except pregnancy; there is no point in detailing them here. Using dysentery as a criterion, I found that in some countries there was a tendency to regard all dysenteries of unknown origin as amebic. Baylet[28] comments on the official figures for Senegal which gave a bacillary-amebic ratio of 0.076, whereas he found Shigella in 77.2% of 219 cases he examined, with *E. dysenteriae* (sic) in 7.8%. His other comments on the situation are, to say the least, scathing.

Amebic disease of the liver was the next syndrome examined. Here too, one came up against misconceptions. The proponents of "amebic hepatitis" could not have appreciated Rogers' Lettsomian lectures[29] or they would not have had to postulate diffuse infiltration of the liver by amebas. This diagnosis became common, even in places where the classical manifestations of amebic invasion are rare. A number of workers (Kean,[30] Roach,[31] Powell et al.[32]) failed to find pathological proof of such a condition. The recent observations by Doxiades et al.[33] have not been acceptable even to those who have seen his material.

Nevertheless the pragmatic label "amebic hepatitis" confused the epidemiological approach, but Elsdon-Dew[34] tabulated the geographical distribution of amebic liver abscess as such. With the limitations set out in his text the table is informative. In general many areas in which amebiasis is said to be rife show a singular lack of reports of liver abscess. The North Coast of Africa is a case in point. It has a bad reputation but though Morocco reported 25,000 cases of amebiasis[35] there has been only one case of liver abscess reported since 1950 (Delanoe[36]). In Africa the main sources of reports of amebic hepatic abscess are Senegal, Nigeria, the Natal coast, and Mozambique.

From Asia Minor most reports of liver abscess and its complications come from Israel, but this may well reflect medical enthusiasm. There is a mass of reports from India, even when those on "amebic hepatitis" are culled. If comparison of early reports with those of recent years is valid there must have been a considerable reduction in the condition. Whether this followed the wholesale use of emetine is not clear.

Thailand and Malaysia report numerous cases, as does Indochina. Of interest is the report by Huard,[37] which contrasts the 17 per 1,000 morbidity in South Vietnam in the 19th century with the 0.7 per 1,000 from 1914 to 1944. No doubt the United States will be encountering repatriate cases, as did the French during their conflict.

No reports on hepatic abscess were available from Japan although fecal surveys give a high incidence of the parasite (Elsdon-Dew[27]). Korea however reports a number of cases. Despite the number of United States cases reported as *ex*-Pacific, there are only three cases from Hawaii and none from Australia. Although odd autochthonous cases are reported from various parts of Europe, the only high incidence noted was in Sicily.

In North America, a notable occurrence was reported in Saskatchewan, Canada, by Eaton[38] and his colleagues. When one recalls that the classical description of Councilman and Lafleur came from Baltimore, it is noteworthy that the condition seems to have disappeared; certainly there were no reports after 1955 for the Northeastern states. For Virginia the only records were in the last century. In Alabama, Hogan[39] reported 16 cases in 50 years. For Georgia the review by Dorrough[40] gives 23 cases in 580,000 admissions over 13 years.

No one seems to have dared to write about amebic hepatic abscess in Louisiana since the monumental work by Ochsner and De Bakey.[41]

Texas seems to have cases imported from Mexico, where the condition is well established (Flores-Barroeta et al.[42]). In Costa Rica there were 13 abscesses in 3,220 autopsies. In Panama, a hotbed judged by fecal surveys (Faust,[43] Jung,[44]), the Gorgas Hospital produced only 50 cases in 25 years (Struve[45]).

The main foci of amebic hepatic abscess in South America seem to be in Colombia, where Cortez-Mendoza[46] found abscess at autopsy in 47 of 728 cases of amebiasis, and Chile (Boero and Shurmann[47]).

If the reported cases of amoebic liver abscess are used as a criterion of invasion by *E. histolytica*, there seem to be relatively few parts of the world where this is common. To summarize: those places seem to be West and Southeast Africa, Southern Asia and the adjacent islands, Mexico, and the western portion of South America.

Of course the use of reported hepatic abscess as a criterion is open to criticism, but it was used *faute de mieux*. Now, of course, we have another parameter in serology (Maddison et al.[48]). As the antibodies arise only as a result of invasion and as they persist after treatment, their prevalence in a community is an index of the frequency of invasion.

Such a technique would be free from the subjectivity of fecal examinations and could be used at some central point. Its use should clarify many misconceptions about the amebic etiology of disease not only in communities and countries but also in those conditions where the causal role of the ameba is questionable.

The defense rests!

*REFERENCES*

1. Ballingall, G.: *Practical Observations on Fever Dysentery and Liver Complaint in India.* Edinburgh, Constable, 1818.
2. Lösch, F.: Massenhaft Entwickelung von Amöben im Dickarm. *Virchow Arch. Path. Anat. 65*:196, 1875.
3. Hlava, J.: *O Uplavici* Z. Böhm Aerzte in Prag (Abstr. Kartulis) 1887.
4. Councilman, W. T. and Lafleur, H. A.: Amebic dysentery. *Johns Hopkins Hosp. Rep. 2*:395, 1891.
5. Casagrandi, O. and Barbagallo, P.: Entamoeba hominis s. Amöeba coli (Lösch) Studio biologico e clinico. *Ann. Igiene 7*:103, 1897.

6. Schaudinn, F.: Untersuchungen uber die Fortpflamzungeiniger Rhizopoden (Vorlaufige Mittheilung) *Arb. Gesundh-Amt.* (Berlin) *19*:547, 1903.
7. Dobell, C.: In: *The Amoebae Living in Man.* London, John Bale, 1919.
8. Huber,—.: Demonstration von Dysenterieamöben, Vereins-Beilage No. 31, p. 267, July 30, 1903, Verein f. innere Med. in Berlin. In: *Deutsche Med. Wochenschr. 29*, 1903.
9. Hartmann, M.: Eine neue Dysenterieamöbe, Entamoeba tetragena (Viereck) syn. Entamoeba africana (Hartmann). *Arch. Schiffs-u. Tropenhyg. 12* (Beih. 5): 117, 1908.

10. Huber,—: Untersuchungen über Amöbendysenterie. *Z. Klin. Med. 67:*202, 1909.

11. Viereck, H.: Studien über die in den Tropen erworbene Dysenterie. *Arch. Schiffs-u. Tropenhyg.* (Beih. I) *11:*1, 1907.

12. Elmassian, M.: Sur une nouvelle espece amibienne chez l'homme, Entamoeba minuta, n.sp. Morphologie—Evolution—Pathogénie. *Zbl. Bakt.* (Orig.) *52: 335,* 1909.

13. Walker, E. L.: The parasitic amoebae of the intestinal tract of man and animals. *J. Med. Res. 17:*379, 1908.

14. Walker, E. L.: A comparative study of the amoebae in the Manila water supply, in the intestinal tract of healthy persons, and in amoebic dysentery. *Philipp. J. Sci.* (B., Trop. Med.) *6:* 259, 1911.

15. Walker, E. L. and Sellards, A. W.: Experimental entamoebic dysentery. *Philipp. J. Sci.* (B., Trop. Med.) *8:* 253, 1913.

16. Kuenen, W. A. and Swellengrebel, N. H.: Die Entamoeben des Menschen und ihre praktische Bedeutung. *Zbl. Bakt.* (Orig.) *71:*378, 1913.

17. Mathis, C. and Mercier, L.: L'amibe de la dysenterie Entamoeba dysenteriae. Councilman, W. T., and Lafleur, H. A., 1891. *Bull. Inst. Pasteur: 14:*641, 1916.

18. Dobell, C.: Amoebic dysentery problem. *J. Trop. Med. Hyg. 21:*115, 1918.

19. Craig, C. F. and Faust, E. C.: *Clinical Parasitology.* Philadelphia, Lea and Febiger, 1943.

20. D'Antoni, J. S.: Concepts and misconcepts in amebiasis. *Amer. J. Trop. Med. 1:*146, 1952.

21. Reichenow, E.: Zur Frage des Sitzes von Entamoeba histolytica im Darm. *Arb. Reischsgesundh. Amt. 57:*136, 1926.

22. Reichenow, E.: Die pathogenetische Bedeutung der Darmprotozoen des Menchen. *Zbl. Bakt.* (Orig.) *122:*195 1931.

23. Hoare, C. A.: The food habits of Entamoeba histolytica in its commensal phase. *Parasitology 42:*43, 1952a.

24. Hoare, C. A.: The commensal phase of Entamoeba histolytica. *Exp. Parasit.*

*1:*411, 1952b.

25. Elsdon-Dew, R.: The Epidemiology of Amoebiasis. *Proc. 7th Int. Cong. Trop. Med. Mal. 2:*268, 1964.

26. Sapero, J., Hankansson, E. G. and Louttit, C. M.: The occurrence of two significantly distinct races of Entamoeba histolytica. *Amer. J. Trop. Med. 22:*191, 1942.

27. Elsdon-Dew, R.: Information available in 1963 on the incidence and geographical distribution of amoebiasis and amoebic liver abscess. *WHO Report MHO/ PA/125,* 1964.

28. Baylet, R. J.: Importance des Shigelloses en pathologie Dakaroise. *Bull. Soc. Path. Exot. 52:*305, 1959.

29. Rogers, L.: Lettsomian lectures on amoebic liver abscess: Its pathology, prevention and cure. Lecture 1. Aetiology and pathology of amoebic liver abscess. *Lancet 1:*463, 1922. Lecture 2. The varieties and treatment of amoebic liver abscess. *Lancet 1:*569, 1922. Lecture 3. The prevention of amoebic liver abscess and the recent reduction in its prevalence and mortality. *Lancet 1:*677, 1922.

30. Kean, B. H.: Amebic hepatitis. Absence of diffuse lesions at autopsy and in biopsies. *Arch. Intern. Med. 96:*667, 1955.

31. Roach, G. G.: The pathology of amoebiasis. *Ann. Inst. Med. Trop.* (Lisboa) *16:* (Suppl. 7) 449, 1959.

32. Powell, S. J., Wilmot, A. J. and Elsdon-Dew, R.: Hepatic amoebiasis. *Trans. Roy. Soc. Trop. Med. Hyg. 53:*190, 1959.

33. Doxiades, T., Candreviotis, N., Tiliakos, M. and Polymeropoulos, I.: Chronic diffuse non-suppurative amoebic hepatitis. *Brit. Med. J. 1:*460, 1961.

34. Elsdon-Dew, R.: The Epidemiology of Amoebiasis. In: *Advances in Parasitology, 6.* London, Acad. Press, 1968.

35. World Health Organization. *Epidem. Vit. Statist. Rep. 11:*97, 1958.

36. Delanoe, G.: Un cas probable de péricardite purulente amibienne. *Bull. Soc. Path. Exot. 53:*787, 1960.

37. Huard, P.: Les abcès du foie au Vietnam. *Med. Trop. 10:*613, 1950.

38. Eaton, R. D. P.: Epidemiological considerations. *Canad. Med. Ass. J. 99:* 706, 1968.
39. Hogan, E. P.: Amebic hepatic abscesses —Prevention and treatment. *Trans. Southern Surg. Ass. 60:322*, 1958.
40. Dorrough, R. L.: Amebic liver abscess. *Southern Med. J. 60:305*, 1967.
41. Ochner, A. and De Bakey, M.: Amebic hepatitis and hepatic abscess. *Surgery 13:* Pt. 1, 460, and Pt. 2, 612, 1943.
42. Flores-Barroeta, F., Nunez, V. and Biagi, F. F.: Observaciones sobre amibiasis en material de autopsia. Estudio de 109 casos. *Prensa Méd. Mex. 24:141*, 1959.
43. Faust, E. C.: In: *Clinical Parasitology*,

Faust and Russell, Philadelphia, Lea and Febiger, 1957, p. 201.
44. Jung., R. C., Garcia-Laverde, A. and Katz, F. F.: In: *Clinical Parasitology*, Faust and Russell, Philadelphia, Lea and Febiger, 1957, p. 989.
45. Struve, E. E.: Amebic abscess of liver. *Calif. Med. 73:178*, 1950.
46. Cortez-Mendoza, E.: Hepatitis amebiana. *Rev. Fac. Med.* (Bogotá) *24:779*, 1956.
47. Boero, D. and Shurmann, R.: Localizaciones extraintestinales de la amibiasis. *Bol. Chil. Parasit. 19:38*, 1964.
48. Maddison, S. E., Powell, S. J. and Elsdon-Dew, R.: The application of serology to the epidemiology of amebiasis. *Amer. J. Trop. Med. 14:554*, 1965.

# AMEBIASIS IN THE UNITED STATES*

KERRISON JUNIPER, JR., M.D.

Department of Medicine
University of Arkansas Medical Center
Veterans Administration Hospital
Arkansas State Hospital
Little Rock, Ark.

## INCIDENCE OF AMEBIASIS

Reviews by Stillwell[1] and Bloomfield[2] indicate that amebiasis was first recognized as a disease of man in Russia by Lösch[3] in 1875 and in Egypt by Kartulis[4] in 1886. The disease was first described in the United States by Osler[5] and Simon[6] in Baltimore in 1890. The first survey of the incidence of the disease in the United States appears to have been in 1913.[7-9] Two factors have made it difficult to arive at a figure representative of the incidence of *Entamoeba histolytica* in the general population of the United States. First, most surveys have not differentiated between the small and large races of *E. histolytica*. Second, most surveys have been performed on groups not representative of the normal general population. Small race *E. histolytica*, now generally accepted as a separate species called *E. hartmanni*, has not been shown to cause disease in man; therefore it must be excluded when the incidence of *E. histolytica* is considered.

Giffin[9] apparently performed one of the earliest parasitological surveys in the United States in 1913 at the Mayo Clinic, Rochester, Minn., where a 4.6% incidence of amebiasis was found. Subsequent surveys have shown rates ranging from 1 to 56% in different populations, the higher figures occuring usually in custodial institutions, especially those for mental illness.[7, 8] In 1942 Faust[10] suggested an incidence of 20%. Probably these high rates were at least in part the result of the factors previously mentioned.

*Presented as part of a *Symposium on Amebiasis* sponsored by The Tropical Disease Center, St. Clare's Hospital, New York, N. Y., and The Merck Company Foundation, Rahway, N. J., held at the Center, September 12, 1970.
This study was supported by U.S. Army Medical Research and Development Command Contract DADA 17-68-C-8148, and National Institutes of Health Training Grant TO1-AM 05314.

McHardy[11] in 1953 and Magath[12] in 1960 disputed the previously accepted amebic infection rates of 10 to 20%. McHardy, who used selected surveys and other sources of information, arrived at an incidence of about 4%. Magath, whose experience at the Mayo Clinic showed infection rates of 1 to 4%, suggested an over-all incidence of less than 1% for the United States.

In 1961 Burrows[13] reevaluated the surveys performed since 1945; he applied a correction based on the known ratio of E. histolytica to E. hartmanni in each area of the United States. He obtained adjusted incidences for E. histolytica (E. hartmanni excluded) of 1% for Alaska, 3 to 6% in the northern United States, and 7 to 10% in the South. More recently Brooke[14] has suggested 5% as a probable estimate of the infection rate in the general population of the country.

## EFFECT OF FOREIGN TRAVEL ON THE INCIDENCE OF AMEBIASIS

Large numbers of servicemen visited countries with high amebic infection rates during World Wars I and II and the conflicts in Korea and Vietnam. Public health authorities feared that the returning infected servicemen would increase the incidence of the disease in the United States. Significant amebic disease did occur in servicemen during World War II, as reflected by Klatskin's observations[15] on troops stationed in India, and the rise in fatal cases documented at the Armed Forces Institute of Pathology and reported by Kean, Gilmore, and Van Stone.[16] Kenamore[17] found amebic dysentery in 10 soldiers returning from tropical theaters of war. Spellberg and Zivin[18] found 34 cases of invasive amebiasis in Illinois veterans during an eight-month period of 1946. At their Veterans Administration Hospital the incidence of amebiasis had been 0.09% before the war and 0.48% in 1946 after the war. Despite these reports in the literature, in 1950 Wright,[19] when he reviewed morbidity and mortality data for the United States, was unable to find evidence of a rise in symptomatic amebiasis caused by the world war.

The recent literature also has reflected an increase in invasive amebiasis since the conflict in Vietnam, as evidenced by the 17 cases of amebic abscess of the liver reported by Sheehy, Parmley, Johnston, and Boyce[20] in 1968, and by sporadic case reports of hepatic abscess from various parts of the country.[21]

Surveys performed on persons returned from the wars usually have failed to show significantly higher infection rates, even though signifi-

121

TABLE I. INCIDENCE OF AMEBIASIS IN TRAVELERS ABROAD

| Report | Group | Number studied | Incidence of amebiasis No overseas service | Overseas service |
|---|---|---|---|---|
| Kofoid et al.[22] | W.W.I Army | 1,200 | 3.0% | 10.8% |
| Jacobs et al.[23] | W.W.II Army | 4,000 | 10.1 | 14-20 |
| Michael[24] | Navy | 1,000 | | 8.9 |
| Marion et al.[25] | Airforce | 1,000 | | 16.8 |
| Conn et al.[26] | Veterans | 3,151 | | 22.7 |
| Lincicome et al.[27] | Veterans | 633 | 2.5 | 4.5 |
| Brooke et al.[28] | Korean veterans | 400 | | 3.0 |
| McQuay[29] | Missionaries | 4,000 | | 3.4 |
| Grossman[30] | Peace Corps | 667 | | 57.0 |

cant amebic disease occurs[22-27] (see Table I). A later survey of Korean war veterans by Brooke, Donaldson, and Brown[28] also failed to show an increased infection rate.

Nonmilitary travel in foreign countries also is increasing and will no doubt become more significant in the future. McQuay[29] examined 4,000 members of missionary families home on furlough and found an *E. histolytica* infection rate of 3.4%, with few symptomatic cases. However, Grossman[30] found 57% of Peace Corps volunteers infected with *E. histolytica* while they were stationed in India; 17% had invasive disease. Thus it appears that although foreign travel so far has not produced much of an increase in the over-all incidence of amebic infection in the United States, invasive amebiasis is being seen in Americans traveling abroad and after their return to this country.

## INVASIVE AMEBIASIS

Although *E. histolytica* apparently can live within the lumen of the colon without causing visible lesions or reactions on the part of the host, when symptoms do occur they are the result of ulceration. The most common symptoms include cramping abdominal pain, diarrhea, and the presence of blood-streaked mucus in the stool. Severe disease may cause loss of weight, low-grade fever, anemia, and leukocytosis. Severe diarrhea with dehydration and electrolyte imbalance is uncommon unless other disease such as bacterial dysentery is present concurrently. When amebomas occur, symptoms of intestinal obstruction may develop and diarrhea can be absent. Liver, lung, and skin are the other organs most often invaded by *E. histolytica*.

In studying amebiasis it is convenient to separate cases into three groups which identify the clinical significance of the infection: asymptomatic, symptomatic noninvasive, and invasive. Diarrhea is the major symptom used in this classification. Asymptomatic patients have no history of diarrhea. When there is a history of diarrhea but no ulcers are found in the rectum, the patient has symptomatic noninvasive disease. Invasive disease is identified by the presence of rectal ulcers from which trophozoites of *E. histolytica* can be obtained in scrapings of the lesions. In rare instances invasive disease is considered present, even though ulcers are not seen, if diarrhea is present and the stools contain blood-streaked mucus from which trophozoites of *E. histolytica* with ingested red blood cells can be demonstrated. Amebomas and extraintestinal amebiasis are classified as invasive disease.

*Endemic disease.* Invasive amebiasis was first reported in the United States in Baltimore[5, 6, 31, 32] and Texas[33] in 1891. Osler,[5] Simon,[6] and Lafleur[32] each reported one patient with amebic dysentery and liver abscess. Councilman and Lafleur[31] reported 14 patients with amebic dysentery, 12 endemic in origin, and provided an excellent description of the organism and the disease. Dock[33] reported 12 patients with amebic dysentery, four of whom also had liver abscess. Osler's textbook of medicine,[34] published in 1893, contained a detailed description of amebic dysentery and hepatic abscess. By 1895 Osler[35] had seen 20 patients with amebic abscess of the liver, and by 1903 Futcher[36] reported the experience of the Johns Hopkins group with 119 cases of amebic dysentery: 96 of the latter cases had been contracted in Maryland and 24% of the patients died. By 1949, when Davis[37] again surveyed the group's experience for the period 1936 to 1946, severe disease was becoming less common, although 296 cases of amebiasis had been seen.

Cases of invasive amebiasis also were reported in significant numbers in Galveston, Texas, in 1914 by Thompson,[38] who described 27 patients with hepatic abscess and a mortality of 19%. Cain, Moore, and Patterson[39] collected 17 cases of amebic abscess of the liver in Galveston between 1956 and 1966. In 1967 May, Lehmann, and Sanford[40] reported 15 patients with liver abscess in Dallas.

The experience of the New Orleans group with invasive amebiasis is well known. In 1933 Gessner[41] recorded 96 cases of amebic abscess of the liver with a mortality of 40% at Charity Hospital. In 1936 Ochsner and DeBakey[42] reported 15 patients with pleuropulmonary amebiasis; they mentioned that at that time 388 cases of amebic dysentery had been seen. In 1951 DeBakey and Ochsner[43] summarized a 20-year experience with 173 cases of amebic abscess of the liver, with a 22% mortality.

Amebic dysentery also was being seen in North Carolina, where Ruffin[44] collected 54 patients, of whom all but four had acquired the disease within the state. By 1946 Smith and Ruffin[45] had seen 134 cases of invasive amebiasis, including 13 with hepatic abscess.

At the Mayo Clinic in 1938 Brown and Hodgson[46] reported 18 patients with amebic abscess of the liver seen over an 18-year period.

In Philadelphia in 1944 Diaz-Rivera and Rasberry[47] presented 32 cases of amebic dysentery collected from one hospital over a 50-year period.

In Memphis in 1960 Webster[48] found that 10 of 48 patients with amebic abscess of the liver had pleuropulmonary involvement.

Recently California has been the source of reports of invasive disease. In 1966 Turrill and Burnham[49] reviewed 66 cases of hepatic amebiasis seen over a 17-year period in Los Angeles. In 1969 Knauer[50] reported 15 patients with amebic abscesses of the liver at several hospitals in San Jose over a 3½-year period; most of these patients had traveled in Mexico and were thought to have acquired their disease there. In 1969 Gaisford and Mark[51] found records on 13 cases of amebic liver abscess seen over a 19-year period in Santa Clara.

In 1967 Dorrough[52] reported 23 patients with amebic abscess collected from hospitals in Atlanta, Ga.

This review indicates that invasive amebiasis has been endemic in the United States and was a significant problem, often with high mortality, during the first half of the 20th century. However, during the past two decades the incidence of invasive amebiasis seems to have declined, although cases of amebic abscess of the liver continue to be reported sporadically in the civilian population.

*Acute outbreaks.* A number of acute outbreaks of invasive amebiasis have occurred since this disease was first recognized in the United States by Osler. In 1917 Craig[53] reported 156 cases of amebic dysentery in soldiers in the El Paso District of Texas. He concluded from his

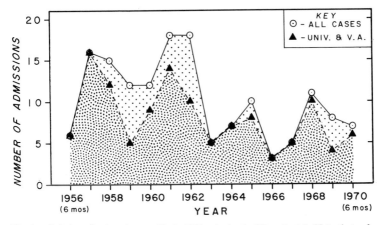

Yearly admissions for invasive amebiasis (153 episodes in 149 patients). Note that only a six-month period is covered in 1956 and 1970.

studies that flies were involved in the spread of the disease.

Three outbreaks have occurred in Chicago. The first, reported in 1927 by Kaplan, Williamson, and Geiger,[54] involved eight cases of amebic dysentery in a hotel where three food handlers were found infected. The second outbreak in 1933 is better known and was reported by Chesley and his associates[55] in 1934. This outbreak included more than 800 cases of amebic dysentery; there were several deaths. The majority of the cases were traced to two hotels where either ice or the water supply had become contaminated with sewage. Hardy and Spector[56] reported a third outbreak at a stockyard fire in 1934, during which a private water supply became contaminated. More than 300 firemen developed diarrhea; six had amebic dysentery, six mild symptomatic amebiasis, and 69 typhoid fever.

A small outbreak of 11 cases of amebic dysentery was reported in Georgia by Secklinger[57] in 1936. A survey showed an amebic infection rate of 12% in that area, but two adjacent areas had incidences of 20 and 39%.

The last outbreak of invasive amebiasis, reported by LeMaistre and associates[58] in 1956, occurred at South Bend, Ind. A private water system at a plant became contaminated with sewage and at least 50% of 1,500

125

TABLE II. INVASIVE AMEBIC DISEASE DURING 14 YEARS IN ARKANSAS
(Number of Patients)

| Source | Invasive colitis | Hepatic abscess | Skin and lung | Total | Deaths No. cases | Percentage |
|---|---|---|---|---|---|---|
| University Hospital | 80 | 18 | 4 | 102 | 4 | 3.9 |
| V.A. Hospital | 9 | 3 | 2 | 14 | 1 | 7.1 |
| Arkansas State Hosp. | 32 | 1 | 0 | 33 | 17 | 52 |
| Total | 121 | 22 | 6 | 149 | 22 | 15 |

employees became infected with *E. histolytica*. There were 31 cases of symptomatic amebiasis and four deaths from the disease.

There is little evidence that acute outbreaks have altered the incidence of amebiasis in the general population. However, in 1934 Freund[59] noted six patients with amebic abscesses of the liver at a Detroit hospital where only 17 such cases had been seen over the preceding five years. In 1943 Hood[60] reported that the incidence of amebiasis at a Chicago hospital increased markedly around the period 1933 to 1934 when the acute outbreak occurred.

*Experience in Arkansas.* I was surprised when I saw six cases of invasive amebiasis during the first six months after joining the faculty at the University of Arkansas Medical Center in Little Rock. Since then I have seen an average of 11 such cases each year (see figure). Over a 14-year period I have been able to document 153 episodes of invasive amebic disease in 149 patients at three local hospitals (Table II). Data from some of these patients have already been reported.[61-65] Strangely, during this same period I have identified only 37 patients with symptomatic noninvasive disease and 54 patients with asymptomatic amebiasis.

The presence of *E. histolytica* has been confirmed from stained smears or tissue sections by members of the Parasitology Section at the National Center for Disease Control in Atlanta in all my cases of intestinal, cutaneous, and pulmonary amebiasis, and in half the cases of hepatic abscess.

The majority of the patients with invasive amebiasis were seen at the University Hospital, but 22% were from the state mental hospital, and 9% from the Veterans Administration Hospital. Nineteen per cent of the 149 patients had extraintestinal disease: 22, hepatic abscess; five, cutaneous amebiasis; and one, pulmonary amebiasis.

Four of the patients with intestinal amebiasis had amebomas, and one, acute amebic appendicitis. Two cutaneous amebic lesions were perianal in location. A third patient developed his skin lesion around a newly created colostomy stoma which was required to relieve an anal stricture. A fourth patient developed a pericecal abscess after a laparotomy for suspected acute appendicitis, and this abscess subsequently ruptured to the abdominal surface and produced a large cutaneous ulcer. The fifth patient developed a large cutaneous amebic lesion on the right flank, presumably from a ruptured superficial liver abscess, although no evidence of hepatic abnormality was present when she was seen.

The patient with pulmonary amebiasis developed a bacteriologically sterile empyema on the right side of his chest after an initial illness thought to be recurrent bacterial pneumonia. Progression of the disease with formation of a bronchopleural fistula necessitated open drainage of the empyema cavity. After nine months of illness, blood serum from this patient happened to be included in a serological screening study of hospital admissions for amebiasis. A strongly positive indirect hemagglutination test suggested the possibility of amebiasis, which had not previously been considered. At this time a history of a mild episode of diarrhea during the first month of his illness was obtained. His liver was normal. E. histolytica was found in his stool, and also in pus draining from the empyema cavity. Antiamebic therapy produced prompt healing.

Although no patients were listed as having amebic abscess of the brain, two patients did develop brain abscesses which might have been amebic in origin but this could not be proved. One patient with invasive colitis was admitted with symptoms of a focal brain lesion, which was found to be a bacteriologically sterile abscess at two craniotomies. He developed bloody diarrhea after the first craniotomy and amebic dysentery was proved. Subsequently he died from uncontrollable hemorrhage from the colon and septicemia. Amebas could not be found in the brain abscess. The patient with cutaneous amebiasis following laparotomy for suspected acute appendicitis developed abscesses in his liver, lung, and brain just prior to his death. The diagnosis of amebiasis was made only at autopsy and amebas were demonstrated in skin, liver, and lung. However, no amebas could be found for certain in the brain abscess.

The over-all death rate of 15% for this series seems high, but the majority of deaths occurred in patients who had mental illnesses. The mortality in the University Hospital and the Veterans Administration Hospital patients was only 4.3%. Of these five deaths, three were patients with liver abscess (one died shortly after admission, a second died despite antiamebic therapy, and a third was not diagnosed prior to autopsy), the fourth had a brain abscess with amebic dysentery accompanied by hemorrhage, and the fifth had unrecognized cutaneous amebiasis and brain abscess.

However, 52% of the mental patients with documented invasive amebiasis died. Only one of these patients had a hepatic abscess; the rest had only severe ulceration of the colon without other complications. Generally death in these patients was totally unexpected since they did not appear to be critically ill. A few patients died before antiamebic therapy could be instituted. However, most seemed to die during the first week of antiamebic therapy, with a peak at three to five days. No specific drug could be related to the deaths since various programs were tried with no alteration of the outcome. This had led me to consider the possibility that death might be related to release of an unusually large amount of amebic antigens with an anaphylactic type of reaction. This high mortality has caused us always to consider mental patients with amebiasis as critically ill, despite absence of findings generally required for this classification.

The unusual amount of invasive amebiasis encountered in Arkansas led to the suspicion of a high incidence of the infection in the state. Consequently Brooke and his associates[66] from the National Center for Disease Control, in cooperation with the Arkansas Department of Public Health, made a survey designed to sample the general population in and near Little Rock in 1963. Single stool specimens were obtained from 357 individuals from four distinct areas with varying sanitary conditions. *E. histolytica* infection rates in the four areas ranged from 1 to 6%, with an average of 3.4%. This survey indicated that an unusually high infection rate did not exist in Arkansas, and therefore was not the explanation for the unusual number of cases of invasive amebiasis being seen.

Two other possibilities were considered. First, the strains of *E. histolytica* encountered in Arkansas might have unusual pathogenicity, thereby causing invasive disease more often. This possibility has not been studied because of the lack of well-developed methods for determining pathogenicity. However, a more likely explanation might be the second possibility: the systematic use of well-developed methods for identifying amebic infection.

Amebiasis is a disease which commonly shows periods of exacerbation and remission without specific antiamebic therapy. Many of our patients had episodes of diarrhea lasting only one to two weeks, followed by a complete remission with healing of rectal ulcers although no antiamebic treatment had been given. The episodes of diarrhea often were infrequent over the course of several years. Since the diarrhea of amebiasis often does disappear without specific treatment, failure to identify the etiologic agent generally leads to a clinical diagnosis of viral enteritis, idiopathic ulcerative colitis, or functional bowel symptoms. Conversely, patients with a diagnosis of chronic amebiasis which has failed to respond to multiple courses of antiamebic therapy rarely if ever are found to have any evidence of amebiasis.

The diagnostic problem is compounded by the fact that antidiarrheal medications, which are present in most family medicine cabinets, generally are tried before patients seek their physician's help. Most of these preparations interfere with demonstration of amebas in the stool. Many patients also receive antibiotics before stool examinations are performed, although the doses generally are sufficient only to suppress the amebic infection without curing it. Many times patients with amebic dysentery have remained undiagnosed because they have received one of the following substances before stool speciments were ceived one of the following substances before stool specimens were examination, antidiarrheal preparations containing heavy metals or alkaline earths, nonabsorbable antacids, sulfonamides, antibiotics, and antiprotozoal drugs. These substances must be discontinued for a period of one to two weeks (probably longer for drugs with a direct effect on amebas) before valid parasitological examinations can be obtained.

I use well-accepted parasitological methods which are described in my chapter in *Gastroenterologic Medicine*,[67] and in the book on laboratory procedures by Melvin and Brooke.[68] However, the manner in which I use these methods is different from that of most clinical laboratories. I encourage immediate sigmoidoscopy after admission as part of the routine workup of patients with diarrhea in order to reduce the possibility that interfering substances will be given to the patient before amebiasis has been excluded. The patient receives *no preparation* for sigmoidoscopy, since this generally reduces the possibility of finding amebas. Any lesions found in the rectum are scraped and the material obtained is used to prepare wet mounts and fixed-stained smears.[67]

My laboratory has performed most of the routine stool examinations for parasites for the University and Veterans Administration hospitals in Arkansas for a number of years, and therefore has encountered most of the problems arising in such work. I soon found it impractical to accept "fresh" stool specimens in a busy laboratory where personnel are not always available to examine such specimens immediately. Another problem encountered with fresh specimens is the inability to have such material examined at night or on weekends, thereby creating difficulty for the physician who may find it necessary to initiate immediate treatment with an interfering substance. Therefore I established one simple system which would handle all hospital and clinic situations, and also allowed for easy follow-up stool examinations at home.

All stool specimens are placed in preservative solutions by the patient or hospital personnel immediately after their passage by the patient. These preserved specimens are then submitted to the laboratory for examination. Fresh stool specimens are not accepted unless specifically requested by the laboratory except in unusual circumstances. We do not follow the practice often used by some parasitologists: that of having the stool specimen submitted fresh and put into the fixing solutions by the laboratory personnel. Short lapses of time between passage of the specimen and placing it in preservative solutions do affect the sharpness of cytologic detail of protozoa, especially the trophozite forms, and can delay a definitive diagnosis. We use PVA (polyvinyl alcohol) and formalin preservative solutions, the pair which has proved so effective in the survey work done by the National Center for Disease Control.[68] Bottles containing the two preservative solutions are kept on the wards and in the clinics. Mailing kits containing a bottle of each fixing solution and directions also are available for use.

## CONCLUSION

I believe that invasive amebiasis is present in other states in which there are large rural areas where wells and outdoor privies are commonly used, especially when flooding occurs frequently. In the preantibiotic era approximately 10 cases of amebic dysentery were found for each case of amebic abscess of the liver in most large series. Today relatively few cases of invasive amebic colitis are being recognized in the United States, despite a low but definite incidence of amebic abscess of the liver. Since invasion of the colon by pathogenic organisms is a prerequisite for development of hepatic abscesses, my explanation for this phenomenon is the frequent nonspecific use of antibiotics, which masks the colonic manifestations of amebiasis and prevents a correct diagnosis but does not cure the infection. Amebic serology, now shown to be highly effective in screening for invasive amebiasis, may help uncover more of these missed amebic infections by enabling the physician to detect suspects and thereby exert more effort to obtain satisfactory parasitological examinations of the stools from these patients.

## ACKNOWLEDGMENTS

I am indebted to Mrs. Rosa Lloyd, Mrs. Cheryl Minshew, Mrs. Harriet Cypert, and Mrs. Linda Roth for assistance in performing the parasitological examinations in my laboratory, and to Drs. Jerome S. Levy and Thomas J. Smith of Little Rock, Dr. Louis P. Good of Texarkana, and Dr. Paul H. Millar, Jr., of Stuttgart for permission to study some of their private patients.

*REFERENCES*

1. Stillwell, G. G.: Amebiasis: Its early history. *Gastroenterology 28:*606-22, 1955.
2. Bloomfield, A. L.: A bibliography of internal medicine: Amebic dysentery. *J. Chron. Dis. 5:*235-52, 1957.
3. Lösch, F.: Massenhafte Entwickelung von Amöben im Dickdarm. *Virch. Arch. Klin. Med. 65:*196-211, 1875.
4. Kartulis, S.: Zur Aetiologie der Dysenterie in Aegypten. *Virch. Arch. Path. Anat. 105:*521, 1886.
5. Osler, W.: On the *Amoeba coli* in dysentery and in dysenteric liver abscess. *Johns Hopkins Hosp. Bull. 1:*53, 1890.
6. Simon, C. E.: Abscess of the liver, perforation into the lung amoeba coli in sputum. *Johns Hopkins Hosp. Bull. 1:* 97, 1890.
7. Craig, C. F. and Faust, E. C.: *Clinical Parasitology,* 5th ed. Philadelphia, Lea & Febiger, 1951, p. 72.
8. Anderson, H. H., Bostick, W. L. and Johnstone, H. G.: *Amebiasis, Pathology, Diagnosis and Chemotherapy.* Springfield, Ill., Thomas, 1953, pp. 15-16.
9. Giffin, H. Z.: Clinical notes on patients from the middle northwest infected with entamebas. *J.A.M.A. 61:*675, 1913.
10. Faust, E. C.: The prevalence of amebiasis in the Western Hemisphere. *Amer. J. Trop. Med. 22:*93-105, 1942.
11. McHardy, G.: Incidence of amebiasis. *Gastroenterology 25:*616-17, 1953.
12. Magath, T. B.: *Entamoeba histolytica:* Its incidence. *Amer. J. Clin. Path. 33:* 441-43, 1960.

13. Burrows, R. B.: Prevalence of amebiasis in the United States and Canada. *Amer. J. Trop. Med. 10:*172-84, 1961.

14. Brooke, M. M.: Epidemiology of amebiasis in the U.S. *J.A.M.A. 188:*519-21, 1964.

15. Klatskin, G.: Observations on amebiasis in American troops stationed in India. *Ann. Int. Med. 25:*773-88, 1946.

16. Kean, B. H., Gilmore, H. R., Jr. and Van Stone, W. W.: Fatal amebiasis: report of 148 fatal cases from the Armed Forces Institutes of Pathology. *Ann. Int. Med. 44:*831-43, 1956.

17. Kenamore, B.: Chronic diarrhea in military personnel returning from the tropics. *Gastroenterology 7:*528-32, 1946.

18. Spellberg, M. A. and Zivin, S.: Amebiasis in veterans of World War II with special emphasis on extra-intestinal complications, including a case of amebic cerebellar abscess. *Gastroenterology 10:* 452-73, 1948.

19. Wright, W. H.: The public health status of amebiasis in the United States, as revealed by available statistics. *Amer. J. Trop. Med. 30:*123-34, 1950.

20. Sheehy, T. W., Parmley, L. F., Jr., Johnston, G. S. and Boyce, H. W.: Resolution time of an amebic liver abscess. *Gastroenterology 55:*26-34, 1968.

21. Juniper, K. Jr.: Amebic abscess of the liver. *Amer. J. Dig. Dis. 14:*290-92, 1969.

22. Kofoid, C. A., Kornhauser, S. I. and Plate, J. T.: Intestinal parasites in overseas and home service troops of the U.S. Army, with especial reference to carriers of amebiasis. *J.A.M.A. 72:*1721-724, 1919.

23. Jacobs, L., Wallace, P. G. and Diamond, L. S.: Survey of intestinal parasites in soldiers being separated from service. *Bull. U.S. Army Med. Dept. 6:* 259-62, 1946.

24. Michael, P.: Intestinal parasitism. A statistical study on 1,000 patients recently returned from Pacific area duty. *Naval Med. Bull. 46:*1589-596, 1946.

25. Marion, D. F. and Sweetsir, F. N.: Amebiasis in military overseas returnees. *Ann. Intern. Med. 24:*186-91, 1946.

26. Conn, H. C., Feldman, P. H. and Taylor, A.: Amebiasis in veterans. *J. Mich. State Med. Soc. 49:*174-81, 1950.

27. Lincicome, D. R., Thiele, W. H. and Capenter, E.: An evaluation of the influence of World War II on the incidence of amebiasis. *Amer. J. Trop. Med. 30:*171-80, 1950.

28. Brooke, M. M., Donaldson, A. W. and Brown, E.: An amebiasis survey in a veterans administration hospital, Chamblee, Georgia, with comparison of technics. *Amer. J. Trop. Med. 3:*615-20, 1954.

29. McQuay, R. M.: Parasitologic studies in a group of furloughed missionaries. I. Intestinal protozoa. *Amer. J. Trop. Med. 16:*154-60, 1967.

30. Grossman, W.: Amebiasis in Peace Corps volunteers. Clinical profile of amebiasis in American volunteers in India. *Amer. J. Gastroenterol. 51:*418-33, 1969.

31. Councilman, W. T. and Lafleur, H. A.: Amoebic dysentery. *Johns Hopkins Hosp. Bull. 2:*395, 1891.

32. Lafleur, H. A.: Dysentery—abscess of liver—*Amoeba coli* in stools and sputum — death — necropsy. *Johns Hopkins Hosp. Bull. 1:*83, 1891.

33. Dock, G.: Observations on the *Amoeba coli* in dysentery and abscess of the liver. *Texas Med. J. 6:*419-31, 1891.

34. Osler, W.: *The Principles and Practice of Medicine.* New York, Appleton, 1893, pp. 132-34.

35. Osler, W.: Abscess of the liver, perforating the lung. *Johns Hopkins Hosp. Bull. 6:*144, 1895.

36. Futcher, T. B.: A study of the cases of amebic dysentery occurring at the Johns Hopkins Hospital. *J.A.M.A. 41:*480-88, 1903.

37. Davis, F. W. Jr.: Amebiasis: Experience in the Johns Hopkins Hospital, 1936-1946. *Amer. J. Med. Sci. 217:*505, 1949.

38. Thompson, J. E.: The pleural and pulmonary complications of tropical abscess of the liver. *Ann. Surg. 59:*891-908, 1914.

39. Cain, C. D., Moore, P. Jr. and Patterson, M.: A ten-year review of amebic abscess of the liver: 1956-1966. *Amer. J. Dig. Dis. 13:*709-17, 1968.

40. May, R. P., Lehmann, J. D. and Sanford, J. P.: Difficulties in differentiating amebic from pyogenic liver abscess. *Arch. Intern. Med. 119:*69-74, 1967.

41. Gessner, H. B.: Abscess of the liver.

*Amer. J. Surg. 20:*683-689, 1933.
42. Ochsner, A. and DeBakey, M.: Pleuropulmonary complications of amebiasis. An analysis of 153 collected and 15 personal cases. *J. Thoracic Surg. 5:*225-58, 1936.
43. DeBakey, M. E. and Ochsner, A.: Hepatic amebiasis. A 20-year experience and analysis of 263 cases. *Int. Abstr. Surg. 92:*209-31, 1951.
44. Ruffin, J. M.: Amebic dysentery in North Carolina. *Amer. J. Dig. Dis. 5:* 153-55, 1938.
45. Smith, C. and Ruffin, J. M.: Amoebic infection of the liver as seen in North Carolina. *Gastroenterology 6:*294-97, 1946.
46. Brown, P. W. and Hodgson, C. H.: Late results in treatment of amebic abscess and hepatitis of the liver. *Amer. J. Med. Sci. 106:*305 13, 1938.
47. Diaz-Rivera, R. S. and Rasberry, E. A.: Amebiasis: Analytical study of the cases admitted to a Philadelphia hospital during the last 5 decades. *Amer. J. Med. Sci. 207:*754-59, 1944.
48. Webster, B. H.: Pleuropulmonary amebiasis. A review with an analysis of ten cases. *Amer. Rev. Resp. Dis. 81:*683-88, 1960.
49. Turrill, F. L. and Burnham, J. R.: Hepatic amebiasis. *Amer. J. Surg. 111:* 424-30, 1966.
50. Knauer, C. M.: Amebic abscess of the liver. Experience with 15 cases in 3½ years in California. *Amer. J. Dig. Dis. 14:*253-61, 1969.
51. Gaisford, W. D. and Mark, J. B. D.: Surgical management of hepatic abscess. *Amer. J. Surg. 118:*317-26, 1969.
52. Dorrough, R. L.: Amebic liver abscess. *Southern Med. J. 60:*305-10, 1967.
53. Craig, C. F.: The occurrence of Entamebic dysentery in the troops serving in the El Paso district from July, 1916, to December, 1916. *Mil. Med. 40:*286-302; 423-434, 1917.
54. Kaplan, B., Williamson, C. S. and Geiger, J. C.: Amebic dysentery in Chicago. Preliminary report of a survey of food handlers following a small outbreak. *J.A.M.A. 88:*977-80, 1927.
55. Chesley, A. J., Craig, C. F., Fishbein, M., Hektoen, L., Magath, T. B., McCoy, G. W., Meleney, H. E., O'Connor,

F. W., Portis, M. and Wolman, A.: Amebiasis outbreak in Chicago. Report of a special committee. *J.A.M.A. 102:* 369-72, 1934.
56. Hardy, A. V. and Spector, B. K.: The occurrence of infestations with *E. histolytica* associated with water-borne epidemic diseases. *Public Health Rep. 50:*323-34, 1935.
57. Secklinger, D. L.: The epidemic of *Entamoeba histolytica* infection in two rural Georgia counties. *Southern Med. J. 29:*472-77, 1936.
58. LeMaistre, C. A., Sappenfield, R. Culbertson, C., Carter, F. R. N., Offutt, A., Black, H. and Brooke, M. M.: Studies of a water-borne outbreak of amebiasis, South Bend, Indiana. I. Epidemiological aspects. *Amer. J. Hyg. 64:*30-45, 1956.
59. Freund, H. A.: Amebic abscess of the liver. Report of cases without previous manifestations of amebiasis. *J.A.M.A. 102:*1550-52, 1934.
60. Hood, M.: The incidence of amebiasis observed at a Chicago hospital over a twelve-year period. *Amer. J. Trop. Med. 23:*327-32, 1943.
61. Juniper, K. Jr., Steele, V. W. and Chester, C. L.: Rectal biopsy in the diagnosis of amebic colitis. *Southern Med. J. 51:*545-53, 1958.
62. Juniper, K. Jr.: Acute amebic colitis. *Amer. J. Med. 33:*377-86, 1962.
63. Juniper, K. Jr.: Acute amebic colitis. *J. Ark. Med. Soc. 55:*362-68, 1959.
64. Juniper, K. Jr.: Treatment of amebiasis. *Mod. Treat. 3:*1016-30, 1966.
65. Juniper, K. Jr.: Acute amebic disease. *J. Ark. Med. Soc. 64:*258-59, 1967.
66. Brooke, M. M., Healy, G. R., Levy, P., Kaiser, R. L. and Bunch, W. L.: A sample survey of selected areas in and near Little Rock, Arkansas, to assess the prevalence of *Entamoeba histolytica. Bull. WHO 92:*813-22, 1963.
67. Juniper, K. Jr.: Parasitic Diseases of the Intestinal Tract. In: *Gastroenterologic Medicine.* Paulson, M., ed. Philadelphia, Lea & Febiger, 1969.
68. Melvin, D. M. and Brooke, M. M.: *Laboratory Procedures for the Diagnosis of Intestinal Parasites.* Public Health Service Publication No. 1969. Washington, D.C., Govt. Print. Office, 1969.

# PATHOGENESIS OF AMEBIASIS *

## R. A. NEAL, Ph.D.

The Wellcome Laboratories of Tropical Medicine
London, England

THIS brief account will deal with *Entamoeba histolytica* only—that is, strains of *E. histolytica* previously classified as the large race. Strains of the small race are now classified as *E. hartmanni*, and are not discussed in the present review. Evidence regarding the specific independence of *E. hartmanni* is fully discussed in a recent review by Elsdon-Dew.[1] A brief reference is made to the *E. histolytica*-like Laredo isolates.

The terminology recommended in the recent WHO Technical Report on amebiasis is used in the paper.[2]

### INTESTINAL AMEBIASIS

*Strain variation.* The laboratory investigations on pathogenicity of *Entamoeba histolytica* commenced with studies on the virulence of different isolates, that is, amebas established in culture from different patients with various clinical signs of amebiasis. The virulence was assessed by determining the infectivity and the degree of ulceration observed in the cecum of the weanling rat. Studies of this type revealed considerable differences of invasiveness between isolates.[3, 4] This type of study has been conducted extensively, the rat being used as the experimental host.[4-8] It was found that the strains from asymptomatic patients were much less virulent than those from symptomatic patients. Similar studies with the guinea pig as the experimental host are less extensive but they also indicate that isolates from asymptomatic patients can have a lower virulence.[9]

In a recent study the invasiveness of *E. histolytica* in the patient was estimated by determining circulating antibody levels, and the virulence of the amebas from each patient was assessed by infecting rats.

---

*Presented as part of a *Symposium on Amebiasis* sponsored by The Tropical Disease Center, St. Clare's Hospital, New York, N. Y., and The Merck Company Foundation, Rahway, N. J., held at the Center, September 12, 1970.

There was a good correlation between the serological titers and virulence to rats.[10]

The amebas which form the inoculum are always accompanied by the bacteria with which they are grown in culture. Therefore the influence of bacteria was studied by several workers. It was found that adding the bacterial flora from virulent strains of *E. histolytica* to avirulent amebas or adding strains of pathogenic bacteria to avirulent amebas did not change the virulence of the isolate of *E. histolytica*.[3, 4, 11] The conclusion from this work is that the amebas alone were responsible for the characteristic virulence of each strain.

This apparent division of isolates into two types led Hoare, following the earlier idea of Brumpt, to propose that *E. histolytica* was divided into two types: avirulent and virulent.[12] However, epidemiological considerations of the wide distribution of these two types, together with the laboratory evidence on the case by which virulence can be changed, show that it is very unlikely that *E. histolytica* can consist of two types that differ only in virulence. In fact the same conclusion was reached independently by Dr. Elsdon-Dew and by me in 1958, that *E. histolytica* could change from the virulent to the avirulent state and vice versa.[13, 14]

The infection of germ-free guinea pigs with *E. histolytica* grown with *T. cruzi* or in the complete absence of other organisms (axenic culture) has thrown further light on the question of the relation between bacteria and amebas. It was found necessary to traumatize the caecal epithelium to enable the amebas to establish local lesions. Such small lesions, however, were very different from the extensive ulceration seen in conventional guinea pigs. Further, none of the germ-free animals died from amebiasis.[15] Germ-free guinea pigs had to be monocontaminated with bacteria such as *Clostridium perfringens* or *Bacterium subtilis*[16] in order to produce a typical reaction to inoculation with bacteria-free amebas. The part played by the bacterium is not yet known. However, it is possible that the bacteria produced a suitable environment (as in redox potential) to support the metabolic integrity of the ameba and may supply a factor in virulence transformation.

At the recent congress on parasitology* Dr. M. Wittner described

---

*Second International Congress on Parasitology, held by the American Society of Parasitologists and the Society of Protozoologists in Washington, D.C., September 6-12, 1970.

135

his studies on incubation of germ-free guinea pigs with axenic amebas. He suggested that the need for direct contact with bacteria might be explained by the occurrence of an episomic-like factor which would be taken up by amebas by phagocytosis.

*Instability of virulence.* Several methods whereby the pathogenicity of *E. histolytica* can be altered have been described. Continued cultivation *in vitro* of virulent strains will result sooner or later in the loss of invasiveness and infectivity to rats or to guinea-pigs.[12, 17, 18] It is possible to increase the virulence of attenuated strains by passage through the liver of a hamster[13] and by direct intestinal passage.[8] However, not all avirulent strains can be made easily invasive by passage through the liver of a hamster.[18]

It has also been found possible to increase virulence by adding cholesterol to cultures of *E. histolytica* or by feeding rats or guinea pigs on this steroid.[18-22] The mechanism of this activity of cholesterol is not yet known, though Gargouri[23] considered its action primarily an irritant to the mucous membrane.

Changes of diet and induced avitaminoses of experimental animals has also shown that more severe infections can be induced.[13] It is not known whether this is reflected in an increased virulence on the part of the ameba or whether such increased virulence is maintained after isolation *in vitro*.

From this discussion it is clear that virulence is an unstable characteristic in *E. histolytica*. On the basis of present evidence, it is my view that amebas are normally avirulent in the intestinal lumen and that, under some stimulus, they change to the invasive form. The stimulus may originate from the host and may result in allowing the amebas to invade the tissues.[24, 25] However, the end result of both mechanisms is that an invasive population of amebas is developed that are different virulent amebas.

*Immunological involvement.* One aspect not yet considered is the immunological reactions between host and parasite in terms of protection of the host. While it is clear that a sterile immunity does not develop, the development of local immunity is not known. The increase of severity of infection when animals are given corticosteroids may have a cellular basis.[26, 27] Antigenic analysis of *E. histolytica* has not yet revealed any clear-cut differences between virulent and nonvirulent amebas.

### HEPATIC AMEBIASIS

It has been shown that *E. histolytica* amebas occur in the liver of the guinea pig. The amebas have wandered from the cecal lesions and are detectable by cultural methods but do not set up definite abscesses.[28] Hepatic injury caused by migratory larvae of the nematode *Toxocara canis* did not promote the development of amebic abscesses.[29] However inoculation of large numbers of amebas via the portal vein in the presence of an existing cecal infection did stimulate the formation of abscesses.[30, 31] Thus it seems that a phenomenon of sensitization may be involved in the development of amebic liver abscess.

### MECHANISM OF INVASION

*Enzymes.* The investigation of enzymes probably related to pathogenic activity has not yielded any clues as to the basis of virulence in *E. histolytica*. Both hyaluronidase and a proteinase closely related to mammalian trypsin have been indentified, but have not been correlated exclusively with virulent isolates.[32] An anomalous observation was the occurrence of carboxypeptidase in avirulent strains but not in virulent strains.

*Toxicity to leukocytes.* Normal leukocytes when in contact with amebas become abnormal within a few minutes. The action of amebas on leukocytes may represent an *in vitro* model for cytotoxic activity of *E. histolytica*.[33, 34]

*Structural observations.* Electron-microscope studies have shown several interesting features. First, in amebas from the human colon a "fuzzy coat" was observed that has not been seen in amebas grown *in vitro*. The function of this structure was not understood and the existence of a mechanism for extracellular secretions of enzymes was not demonstrated.[35]

The second structural feature was described by Eaton, Meerovitch, and Costerton.[36] During studies of the behavior of *E. histolytica* in tissue-cell culture it was observed that *E. histolytica* appeared to kill cells by contact. Ultrastructural observations showed the presence of cup-shaped lysosome structures on the surface of the ameba. In the center of the organelle is a projection which may act as a trigger mechanism. A filamentous structure was also observed in amebas from experimentally infected rats but not in amebas from culture (Rondanelli et al.[37]). The authors thought that the structures might be related

137

to ameboid movement but perhaps they are adaptations to living in tissue.

Follow-up studies on these structures are awaited with interest.

## E. histolytica-LIKE AMEBAS

These amebas are distinguished from true E. histolytica by their ability to grow at relatively low temperatures—at about 26°C.[38] There are further differences in response to hypertonic solutions, antigenic composition, sensitivity to drugs, and biochemistry (free amino acid composition and fructokinase).

All known strains of these amebas were isolated from asymptomatic patients and were avirulent in experimental animals. All were isolated in the United States.

## COMMENT

It is clear that there is still no definite information as to the underlying basis of pathogenesis of E. histolytica, although there are a number of interesting leads which may develop during the next few years. One of the problems is the difficulty of studying the amebas, since we do not have a convenient simple model for the determination of invasiveness. The infection of laboratory animals is still necessary.

### REFERENCES

1. Elsdon-Dew, R.: The epidemiology of amoebiasis. *Adv. Parasit.* 6:1-62, 1968.
2. *Amoebiasis.* WHO Tech. Rept. Ser. 1969. No. 421, pp. 1-52.
3. Frye, W. W. and Shaffer, J. G.: Experimental pathology of amebiasis. *Proc. 4th Int. Congr. Trop. Med. Malar.,* 1075-87, 1948.
4. Neal, R. A.: Virulence in *Entamoeba histolytica. Trans. Roy. Soc. Trop. Med. Hyg. 45:*313-19, 1957.
5. Singh, B. N., Mathew, S., Sharma, R. and Saxena, V.: Virulence of strains of Entamoeba histolytica from human carrier and acute cases in rats. *J. Sci. Indust. Res. 17C:*201-03, 1958.
6. Sarkisyan, M.A. and Vaskanyan, K. M.: Data of an experimental study of strains of *Entamoeba histolytica* isolated from patients with amoebiasis and from healthy carriers. *Med. Parasitol. Parasit. Dis. 35:*357-62, 1966.
7. Mizgireva, M. F.: Comparative virulence of *Entamoeba histolytica,* isolated from patients and different groups of carriers. *Med. Parasitol. Parasit. Dis. 35:*201-04, 1966.
8. Healy, G. R. and Gleason, N. N.: Studies on the pathogenicity of various strains of *Entamoeba histolytica* after prolonged cultivation, with observations on strain differences in the rats employed. *Amer. J. Trop. Med. 15:*204-99, 1966.
9. Kasprzak, W.: Biological characteristics of the strains of *Entamoeba histolytica* from the carriers in Poznan Palatinate. *Acta Parasit. Polon. 9:*211-230, 1961.
10. Neal, R. A., Robinson, G. L., Lewis, W. P. and Kessel, J. F.: Comparison of

clinical observations on patients infected with *Entamaeba histolytica,* with serological titres of their sera and virulence of their amoebae to rats. *Trans. Roy. Trop. Med. 62:*69-75, 1968.

11. Sarkisyan, M. A.: On the role of the bacterial flora in the reproduction of experimental amoebiasis. *Med. Parasitol. Parasit. Dis. 36:*715-721, 1967.

12. Hoare, C. A.: The enigma of host-parasite relations in amebiasis. *Rice Inst. Pamphl. 45:*23-35, 1958.

13. Neal, R. A.: The pathogenicity of *Entamoeba histolytica. Proc. 6th Int. Congr. Trop. Med. Malar. 3:*350-59, 1958.

14. Elsdon-Dew, R.: The host parasite relationship in amoebiasis. *S. Afr. Med. J. 32:*89-92, 1958.

15. Phillips, B, P., Wolfe, P. A. and Bartgis, I. L.: Studies on the ameba-bacteria relationship in amebiasis. 11. Some concepts on the etiology of the disease. *Amer. J. Trop. Med. 7:*392-99, 1958.

16. Phillips, B. P. and Gorstein, F.: Effects of different bacteria on the pathology of enteric amebiasis in monocontaminated guinea-pigs. *Amer. J. Trop. Med. 15:*863-68, 1966.

17. Biagi, F. F. and Marvin, A. G.: El poder patogeno de *Entamoeba histolytica* como caracteristica inestable. *Prensa Med. Mex. 29:*15-16, 1964.

18. Carneri, I. de: Studi sulla virulenza de *Entamoeba histolytica.* I. Variazioni ciceiche della virulenza di un ceppo de *Entamoeba histolytica* nell' infezione intestinale del ratto albino in seguito a passaggi serioli in vitro e nel fegato *di Cricetus auratus. Riv. Parassit. 19:* 7-20, 1958.

19. Sharma, R.: Effect of cholesterol on the growth and virulence of *Entamoeba histolytica. Trans. Roy. Soc. Trop. Med. Hyg. 53:*278-81, 1959.

20. Singh, B. N.: Effect of cholesterol on the virulence of *Entamoeba histolytica* in rats. *J. Sci. Indust. Res. 18C;* 166-169, 1959.

21. Biagi, F. F., Robledo, E., Servín, H. and Martuscelli, A.: The effect of cholesterol on the pathogenicity of *Entamoeba histolytica. Amer. J. Trop. Med. 11:*333-340, 1962.

22. Biagi, F. F., Robledo, E., Servín, H. and Marván, G.: Influence of some steroids in the experimental production of amoebic hepatic abscess. *Amer. J. Trop. Med. 12:*318-20, 1963.

23. Gargouri, M.: L'utilisation de cholesterol dans l'amibiase experimentale du cobaye. *Ann Parasit.* (Paris) *42:*399-402, 1967.

24. Kasprzak, W.: Variation between strains of *Entamoeba histolytica. Abst. 8th Cong. Trop. Med. Malar.,* p. 248, 1968.

25. Mizgireva, M. F.: The variability of the virulent properties of *Entamoeba histolytica. Med. Parasitol. Parasit. Dis. 35:*673-676, 1966 b.

26. Teodorovic, S., Ingalis, J. W. and Greenberg, L.: Effects of corticosteroids on experimental amoebiasis. *Nature 197:*86-87, 1963.

27. Lapasco, Gh., Silard, R. and Soresco, A.: Recherches experimentales sur la reacquisition de la pathogenicite d'une souche d'*Entamoeba dysenteriae. Arch. Roum. Path. Exp. Microbiol. 27:*269-74, 1968.

28. Rees, C. W., Taylor, D. J. and Reardon, L. V.: The presence of *Entamoeba histolytica* in the liver of guinea-pigs with experimental intestinal amebiasis. *J. Parasit. 40:*390-91, 1954.

29. Krupp, I. M.: Amebic invasion of the liver of guinea-pigs infected with the larvae of a nematode *Toxacara canis. Exp. Parasit. 5:*421-26, 1956.

30. Maegraith, B. G. and Harinasuta, C.: Experimental amoebic infection of the l·ver in guinea-pigs. 11. Abscess formation in animals with persistent lesions. *Ann. Trop. Med. Parasit. 48:*434, 1954.

31. Biagi, F. F. and Beltran, H. F.: Amibiasis un reto a la comprensíon de los mecanismos patogenicos. *Gac. Med. Mex. 97:*71-73, 1967.

32. Jarumilinta, R. and Maegraith, B. G.: Enzymes of *Entamoeba histolytica. Bull. WHO 41:*269-73, 1969.

33. Jarumilinta, R. and Knakolfer, F.: Hyaluronidase activity in stock cultures of *Entamoeba histolytica. Ann. Trop. Med. Parasit. 54:*118-28, 1964.

34. Artigas, J., Otto, I. and Kawada, M. E.: Acción de *Entamoeba histolytica* sobre

leucocitos polimonfonudearis humanos vivos. *Bol. Chil. Parasit. 21*:114-18, 1966.

35. El-Hashmid, W. and Pittman, F.: Ultrastructure of *Entamoeba histolytica* trophozoites obtained from the colon and from *in vitro* cultures. *Amer. J. Trop. Med. 19*:215-26, 1970.

36. Eaton, R. D. P., Meerovitch, E. and Costerton, J. W.: A surface active lysosome in *Entamoeba histolytica. Trans.*

*Roy. Soc. Trop. Med. Hyg. 63*:678-80, 1969.

37. Rondanelli, E. G., Carosi, G., Gerna, G. and De Carneri, I.: Sul reperto di corpi filamentosi paranucleari in *Entamoeba histolytica in vivo.* Richerche microelettroniche. *Boll. Inst. Sieroter* (Milan) *47*:401-05, 1968.

38. Goldman, M.: Entamoeba histolytica-like amoebae occurring in man. *Bull. WHO 40*:355-64, 1969.

# THERAPY OF AMEBIASIS*

## S. John Powell, M.D.

Professor of Tropical and Preventive Medicine
Amoebiasis Research Unit
University of Natal
Durban, South Africa

## Introduction

A MEBIASIS is a readily curable condition which responds promptly and nearly always completely to correct management. The commonest cause of the failure of treatment is faulty diagnosis due to the incorrect identification of *Entamoeba histolytica*. In many other instances, however, it results from erroneous assumptions regarding the pathogenicity of the parasite. This leads to treatment that is frequently inadequate, at other times excessive and, perhaps even more often, entirely irrelevant. Such assumptions have resulted in misleading claims of the efficacy of various amebicides and in neglect of the cardinal principle that treatment should be directed at the three possible sites where *E. histolytica* may exist. These sites are the bowel lumen, the intestinal wall and, systemically, particularly the liver.

The story of drug treatment in amebiasis reflects the background of changing concepts of the nature and pathogenicity of *E. histolytica*.

Modern knowledge of clinical amebiasis dates from the latter part of the last century, when the disease was clearly recognized as invasive, presenting with the often fatal conditions of amebic dysentery and hepatic abscess. Ipecacuanha had long been used in treatment[1] but the first and enduring landmark in treatment was the introduction of emetine hydrochloride by Rogers in 1912.[2] This drug proved to be lifesaving and, although limited by toxicity, it has remained universally successful wherever severe amebiasis is encountered. However, despite its efficacy as a tissue amebicide, it frequently fails to eradicate amebas from the lumen of the bowel, and recurrence of symptoms is common. This is a major reason why amebiasis has gained the reputation of being a chronic, relapsing condition. In fact, resistance is not an inherent

*Presented as part of a *Symposium on Amebiasis* sponsored by The Tropical Disease Center, St. Clare's Hospital, New York, N. Y., and The Merck Company Foundation, Rahway, N. J., held at the Center, September 12, 1970.

property of the ameba and relapse is due to the limitations of many amebicides. Emetine hydrochloride alone is never adequate.

Oral preparations of emetine were introduced to achieve greater activity in the bowel lumen,[3] and they have yielded high rates of cure in intestinal amebiasis.[4] The combination of emetine hydrochloride with emetine bismuth iodide is still found adequate by many experienced physicians.[5] It is, however, an unpleasant medication and, in our experience, it regularly causes diarrhea. Nausea and vomiting are also frequent.

Shortly after World War I the view became prevalent, particularly in the United States,[6, 7] that *E. histolytica* was an obligate pathogen which always invaded the tissues. Since infection was known to be common in temperate regions this implied that there were vast numbers of individuals in need of treatment. Consequently during the next two decades impetus was given to the development of.drugs which would remove these amebas from the bowel. The number of such luminal amebicides produced is too numerous to list but prominent among them were oral arsenicals and quinoline derivatives. More modern preparations have appeared since World War II, of which diloxanide furoate is a notable example.[8] All are capable of eradicating lumen-dwelling amebas to a varying degree and have enjoyed a vogue in temperate countries for the treatment of symptomless and mildly symptomatic bowel infections, but all have been found inadequate where amebiasis is associated with a significant degree of tissue invasion.[9]

At this point it is relevant to digress in order to consider the problem of treating chronic bowel infections. Although the concept of *E. histolytica* as an obligate pathogen is no longer universally accepted[10] it continues to tempt practitioners to ascribe a wide range of symptoms to presence of the ameba. When specific treatment has failed to bring relief the drug is blamed. Should repeated courses of amebicides then be given for the long-since exterminated, innocent, and probably commensal amebas? Both practitioner and patient are often left with the conviction that "amebiasis" is a chronic and incurable condition. To achieve cure in such instances, education of the physician is more effective than amebicides for the patient. It is a sound general rule that when symptoms have failed to respond to a reputable amebicide the diagnosis should be questioned and search made elsewhere for the cause of the patient's complaints. Serological tests are invaluable in ascertaining if symptoms are likely to have been caused by *E. histolytica* but there is some danger that the tests and not the patient will be treated. It should also be borne in mind that apparent response to an amebicide is not diagnostic of amebiasis. Many patients with other disorders, often of a psychosomatic nature, may appear to respond, although this is usually only temporary.

Nowadays the consensus is that in the vast majority of infected subjects *E. histolytica* is merely a commensal living within the lumen of the bowel.[11] In most temperate regions infected persons are extremely unlikely ever to suffer significant invasion of the tissue that results in disease. However, this can occur on rare occasions; thus many feel that treatment of such symptomless cystpassers or coincidental infections is justified. Others are concerned that this attitude opens the floodgates of indiscriminate treatment, encouraging the development of bowel neuroses and the neglect of other organic disease. Since it has not yet been shown that the presence of *E. histolytica* is ever actively beneficial, strong views against treatment under these circumstances are hardly tenable although there are greater priorities in medicine. But if amebicides are given, neither the physician nor patient should be in any doubt of the limited objectives of the therapy.

In regions where there is much invasive amebiasis commensal infections are also common. However, tissue invasion may be symptomless and, presumably, the chance of its taking place is greater in endemic areas. Moreover in such regions symptomless carriers may be the cause of invasive infections in others. Hence where invasive amebiasis is endemic the case for treating symptomless or possibly coincidental infections is stronger although the undesirable results of indiscriminate treatment are perhaps greater. "Amebaphobia" flourishes particularly in places where true invasive amebiasis is present to lend a background of authenticity to diagnostic claims that would otherwise be unconvincing if not absurd.

The end of World War II heralded the era of antibiotics in amebiasis. In 1945 Hargreaves[12] demonstrated the value of penicillin and sulphonamides in amebic dysentery. Soon after this it became evident that the tetracyclines were the most effective of all, acting on *E. histolytica* apparently indirectly by modifying the bacterial flora of the bowel.[13-16] The original tetracyclines remain the antibiotics of choice but relapse may occur after apparent cure, and no tetracycline is of value in hepatic amebiasis.[17]

Table I. AMEBIC DYSENTERY: RESULTS OF TREATMENT AND SITE OF ACTION OF AMEBICIDES

| Therapy | Bowel lumen | Bowel wall | | Percentage cure |
|---|---|---|---|---|
| Emetine HCL or Dehydroemetine | − | + | + | 30-50 |
| Emetine HCL + E.B.I. | + | + | + | 92 |
| Luminal amebicides | + | − | − | 20-50 |
| Oral tetracycline | + | + | − | 97 |
| Chloroquine | − | − | + | 10 |
| Tetracycline + luminal amebicide + chloroquine | + | + | + | 98 |
| Tetracycline + luminal amebicide + emetine HCL or dehydroemetine | 86 | + | + | + |

In contrast Conan[18] showed that chloroquine was effective in amebic abscess of the liver although it has little activity in the bowel. As a less toxic alternative to emetine the drug achieved wide usage but it is inferior.[19, 20] Nevertheless, it is of value as a supplementary medication.[21]

The synthetic preparation dehydroemetine appeared in 1959.[22] Because of more rapid excretion and a more favorable liver-heart concentration ratio, it was hailed as an advance on natural emetine.[23] While some doubt has been cast on claims of reduced toxicity,[24] in practice the drug is a satisfactory alternative to emetine.[25] However, it possesses precisely the same limitations.

Until approximately five years ago these were the major drugs available for treatment. Our findings in 20 years of controlled trials in Durban are summarized in the two accompanying tables.

No single drug was adequate and the selective actions of all were a source of confusion, but when they are used in correct combination excellent rates of cure can be obtained. Although it is by no means essential that these preparations should be entirely abandoned, recent developments have lessened their value for, compared to the newest drugs, such combinations are more complicated and tedious to use, and some occasionally exhibit toxicity.

In 1964 a preliminary report of the effect of niridazole in amebic abscess of the liver[26] led to the introduction of a new series of compounds in therapy. It was soon demonstrated that niridazole alone was

TABLE II. AMEBIC LIVER ABSCESS: RESULTS OF TREATMENT

| Treatment* | Percentage cure |
|---|---|
| Emetine 65 mg. × 10 days | 88 |
| Emetine 65 mg. (2 courses) | 100 |
| Dehydroemetine 80 mg. × 10 days | 88 |
| Dehydroemetine 80 mg. (2 courses) | 89 |
| Chloroquine × 28 days | 71 |
| Emetine 65 mg. + chloroquine | 98 |
| Dehydroemetine 80 mg. + chloroquine | 100 |

*In all instances a luminal amebicide was also given and, when concomitant dysentery was present, tetracycline was added.

capable of curing both intestinal and hepatic amebiasis, but an undesirable degree of toxicity was evident.[27]

It was not long, however, before another nitroheterocyclic compound was found to yield even better results. This is the nitroimidazole derivative metronidazole. The drug had been safely and widely used since 1959 for the treatment of trichomoniasis, but the first successful clinical trials in amebiasis did not appear until 1966.[28] Since then favorable results of numerous and extensive trials, particularly in invasive amebiasis, have been reported.[29, 30] In appropriate dosage metronidazole has proved equally effective in childhood amebiasis.[31-33] At present metronidazole is unique as a safe, single, direct-acting amebicide with activity at all sites. It is the treatment of choice in most forms of amebiasis.

Much of our most recent work on metronidazole in Durban has been concerned with duration of the treatment. The almost traditional viewpoint that amebiasis is often a chronic and relapsing condition led to the belief that prolonged and often repeated courses of amebicides were necessary to achieve cure. We believe that this is really a reflection on the adequacy of the drugs and that if a sufficient concentration of an effective preparation can be achieved duration of treatment can be short. We find that a single large dose of 2.0 to 2.4 gr. of metronidazole is capable of curing a high proportion of patients with amebic dysentery or hepatic abscess. If this dose is repeated on a second day the rate of cure is higher and appears adequate in many regions. In the severe cases encountered in Durban three such doses yield results which are similar to those obtained by our previously recommended, optimal five-day course.[34, 35] There is now a choice of regimens available.

.It is important to realize that metronidazole is highly absorbed; hence smaller doses are effective in the tissues than in the intestinal lumen. Good results have been reported in symptomless cyst-passers and mild dysentery,[36] but the temptation to use too small a dosage should be avoided. Newer nitroheterocyclic compounds are likely to appear in the near future, but it must be borne in mind that laboratory evidence of increased activity is liable to be offset by increased absorption. Higher blood and tissue levels will result but the concentration in the intestine may remain inadequate.

For detailed accounts of the modern management of various forms of amebiasis and its complications reference should be made to other publications,[9, 37-40] but our routine drug therapy can be summarized as follows:

*Symptomless intestinal amebiasis.* There is a wide choice of luminal amebicides. Diloxanide furoate, o.5 gr. thrice daily orally for 10 days, is satisfactory. Alternatively metronidazole, 400 to 800 mg. thrice daily for 5 days, may be used.

*Chronic nondysenteric intestinal amebiasis.* Mild cases with minimal or no invasion of tissue may respond to luminal amebicides but as a general rule treatment should be as for amebic dysentery.

*Amebic dysentery.* Metronidazole, either a single dose of 2.0 to 2.4 gr. on three successive days, or 800 mg. thrice daily for 5 days.

*Hepatic amebiasis.* Metronidazole, 400 mg. thrice daily for five days, or a single dose of 2.0 to 2.4 gr. on two or three successive days. While small abscesses repond to drugs alone, closed aspiration remains an essential part of management in many cases. The indications and technique for this procedure are well described.[9, 37, 40-41] Nevertheless, inadequate drainage is the commonest reason for failure of treatment and relapse.

*Relapse in intestinal amebiasis.* Because of the tendency of many drugs to convert patients to a temporary state of symptomless cyst-passing with eventual relapse, examination of stools, including a concentration technique, should be performed one month after completing treatment and, if possible, again after two months. Where circumstances permit, search should be made for a source of reinfection in all adequately treated patients who suffer relapse. Not infrequently the source is a member of the same household with a symptomless infection.

*Prophylaxis.* Diarrhea is a common affliction among visitors to warm climates. It has been repeatedly shown that *E. histolytica* is not a significant cause of this condition, yet large quantities of luminal amebicides are still consumed for both prophylaxis and treatment. It may be, although I doubt it, that some of the drugs are of value in preventing such traveler's diarrhea, but it needs to be stressed that this is not amebiasis.

In regions of endemic amebiasis there is always the possibility that an individual may become infected but the chance is small. In Durban, where invasive amebiasis is highly endemic in the black community, both infection and disease are rare in whites. To accept the recommendation that such individuals, whether resident or visitant, should take prophylactic amebicides is absurd. It is a gross exaggeration to suggest that the need for prophylaxis against amebiasis is in any way similar to that for protection against a condition such as malaria.

The only solid indication for prophylaxis that I can envisage is in sudden outbreaks of invasive amebiasis. These are rare but they occur in association with contamination of drinking water by sewage.

## CONCLUSIONS

The advent of metronidazole has greatly simplified therapy and has proved of particular value in the treatment of invasive amebiasis. However, the drug should not be looked upon as a simple and safe cure-all to be used indiscriminately in place of accurate diagnosis. Although the necessity to resort to the older amebicides has diminished, they need not be entirely abandoned. Indeed, in some instances parenteral emetine preparations remain essential and life-saving. Nor should the availability of metronidazole cause us to neglect such basic principles of management as fluid and electrolyte replacement in dysentery and the need for aspiration in hepatic abscess.

In the near future we can expect to see the introduction of several compounds similar to metronidazole. In correct dosages, I believe some will be found effective but it is likely to prove very difficult, if not impossible, to single them out on a basis of individual merit.

REFERENCES

1. Docker, E. S.: On the treatment of dysentery by the administration of large doses of ipecacuanha. *Lancet 2:*113, 1858.
2. Rogers, L.: The rapid cure of amoebic dysentery and hepatitis by hypodermic injections of soluble salts of emetine. *Brit. Med. J. 1:*1424, 1912.
3. Du Mez, A. G.: Two compounds of emetine which may be of service in the treatment of entamoebiasis. *Philipp. J. Sci. 10:*73, 1915.
4. Manson-Bahr, P.: Amoebic dysentery and its effective treatment. A critical study of 535 cases. *Brit. Med. J. 2:*255, 1941.
5. Woodruff, A. W.: Amoebicides. *Practitioner 183:*92, 1959.
6. Craig, C. F.: *Manual of Parasitic Protozoa of Man.* Philadelphia, Lippincott, 1926, p. 569.
7. Faust, E. C.: Amebiasis in New Orleans population as revealed by autopsy examination of accident cases. *Amer. J. Trop. Med. 21:*35, 1941.
8. Woodruff, A. W. and Bell, S.: Clinical trials with Entamide Furoate and related compounds. *Trans. Roy. Soc. Trop. Med. Hyg. 54:*389, 1960.
9. Powell, S. J.: Drug therapy of amoebiasis. *Bull. WHO 40:*953, 1969.
10. *Amoebiasis.* Report of a WHO expert committee. WHO Tech. Rep. Series No. 421, 1969, p. 8.
11. Alvarez, W. C.: Amebaphobia. *Proc. Mayo Clin. 10:*84, 1935.
12. Hargreaves, W. H.: Chronic amoebic dysentery. A new approach to treatment. *Lancet 2:*68, 1945.
13. McVay, L. V., Laird, R. L. and Sprunt, D. H.: Preliminary report of the successful treatment of amebiasis with Aureomycin. *Science 109:*590, 1949.
14. Armstrong, T. G., Wilmot, A. J. and Elsdon-Dew, R.: Aureomycin and amoebic dysentery. *Lancet 2:*10, 1950.
15. Most, H. and Van Assendelft, F.: Laboratory and clinical observations on the effect of Terramycin in the treatment of amebiasis. *Ann. N. Y. Acad. Sci. 53:*427, 1950.
16. Wilmot, A. J. A comparison of puromycin and tetracycline and its deriva-

tives in amebiasis. *Antibiotics Annual.* New York p. 319, 1955-56.
17. Powell, S. J. MacLeod, I. N., Wilmot, A. J. and Elsdon-Dew, R.: Further drug trials in acute amoebic dysentery: demethylchlortetracycline, methacycline, ampicillin and chlorhydroxquinoline. *Trans. Roy. Soc. Trop. Med. Hyg. 59:* 709, 1965.
18. Conan, N. J.: Chloroquine in amebiasis. *Amer. J. Trop. Med. 28:*107, 1948,
19. Harinasuta, C. A.: Comparison of chloroquine and emetine in the treatment of amoebic liver abscess. *Indian Med. Gaz. 86:*137, 1951.
20. Wilmot, A. J. Powell, S. J. and Adams, E. B.: The comparative value of emetine and chloroquine in amebic liver abscess. *Amer. J. Trop. Med. 7:*197, 1958.
21. Wilmot, A. J., Powell, S. J. and Adams, E. B.: Chloroquine compared with chloroquine and emetine combined in amebic liver abscess. *Amer. J. Trop. Med. 8:*623, 1959.
22. Brossi, A., Baumann, N., Chopard-ditJean, L. H., Würsch, J., Schneider, F. and Schneider, O.: Syntheseversuche in der Emetine-Reihe 4. Mitteilung Racemisches 2-Dehydro-emtin. *Helv. Chim. Acta. 42:* 772, 1959.
23. Schwartz, D. E. and Herrera, J.: Comparative pharmakinetic studies of dehydroemetine and emetine in guinea pigs using spectrofluorometric and radiometric methods. *Amer. J. Trop. Med. 14:*78, 1965.
24. Johnson, P. and Neal, R. A.: The amoebicidal activity and toxicity of natural emetine, (+) —2— dehydrometine and (−) —2— dehydrometine. *Ann. Trop. Med. Parasit. 62:*455, 1968.
25. Powell, S. J.: Dehydrometine in the treatment of invasive amoebiasis. *Proc. Eighth Internat. Cong. Trop. Med. Malaria.* Teheran, 1968.
26. Kradolfer, F. and Jarumilinta, R.: A new systemically active amoebicide. Ciba 32644-Ba. *Proc. 1st Internat. Cong. Parasit.* Rome, 1966, p. 397.
27. Powell, S. J., Wilmot, A. J. and Elsdon-Dew, R.: The use of niridazole alone and in combination with other amoebi-

cides in amoebic dysentery and amoebic liver abscess. *Ann. N. Y. Acad. Sci. 160:* 749, 1969.

28. Powell, S. J. MacLeod, I., Wilmot, A. J. and Elsdon-Dew, R.: Metronidazole in amoebic dysentery and amoebic liver abscess. *Lancet 2:*1329, 1966.
29. *Ind. Practit.* (special number on amoebiasis and giardiasis) *21:*613, 1968.
30. *Med. Today* (special number on amoebiasis today) *3:*1, 1969.
31. Watson, C. E., Leary, P. M. and Hartley, P. S.: Amoebiasis in Cape Town children. *S. Afr. J. Med. Sci. 44:*419, 1970,
32. Rubidge, C. J., Scragg, J. N. and Powell, S. J.: Treatment of children with acute amoebic dysentery. *Arch. Dis. Child. 45:*196, 1970.
33. Scragg, J. N. and Powell, S. J.: Metronidazole and niridazole combined with dehydroemetine in the treatment of children with amoebic liver abscess. *Arch. Dis. Child. 45:*193, 1970.
34. Powell, S. J., Wilmot, A. J. and Elsdon-

Dew, R.: Single and low dosage regimens of metronidazole in amoebic dysentery and amoebic liver abscess. *Ann. Trop. Med. Parasit. 63:*139, 1969.
35. Powell, S. J.: Clinical aspects of amoebiasis. *Med. Today 4:* 57, 1970.
36. Khambatta, R. B.: Metronidazole in chronic intestinal amoebiasis. *Ann. Trop. Med. Parasit. 62:*139, 1968.
37. Powell, S. J.: Amebiasis. In: *Current Therapy,* Conn, H. F. ed. Philadelphia, Saunders, 1969, p. 3.
38. Wilmot, A. J.: Intestinal amoebiasis. *Practitioner 203:*634, 1969.
39. Powell, S. J.: Management of amoebiasis. In: *The Management and Treatment of Tropical Diseases,* Maegraith, B. G. and Gillis, H. M., eds. Oxford, Blackwell, 1970.
40. Wilmot, A. J.: *Clinical Amoebiasis.* Oxford, Blackwell Scient. Publ., 1962, p. 94.
41. Powell, S. J.: Amoebic liver disease. *Ghana Med. J. 8:*100, 1969.

# LABORATORY DIAGNOSIS OF AMEBIASIS*

GEORGE R. HEALY, Ph. D.

Chief, Helminthology and Protozoology Unit
Center for Disease Control
Atlanta, Ga.

THE laboratory diagnosis (that is, the recovery and identification) of *Entamoeba histolytica* is a topic normally reported in publications concerned with the diagnosis of intestinal parasitic infections in general. There has been an increased awareness of the importance of proper diagnostic techniques in parasitology.

These techniques were once merely discussed in appendices of books on tropical medicine or parasitology but are now treated as a distinct and separate subject. Among the books published in recent years are those by Burrows,[1] and by Markell and Voge,[2] there is also a recent Public Health Service (PHS) bulletin by Melvin and Brooke,[3] and an excellent color atlas by Spencer and Monroe.[4]

Few books or monographs have specifically dealt with the laboratory diagnosis of amebiasis, those of Anderson et al.,[5] Faust,[6] Brooke,[7] and a PHS[8] manual are the principal ones of the past 10 years. In contrast, short articles on the laboratory diagnosis of amebiasis have been published by a variety of authors in a number of journals for many years, attesting to the continued importance of the subject[9-20] and the necessity for periodic review. Since it is nearly impossible to consider all facets of laboratory diagnosis in one report, only certain aspects of the subject will be highlighted here.

To the layman, the term "amebiasis" may mean very little. On the other hand, the statement "amebic dysentery" immediately calls to mind for most people exactly what amebiasis is in its classic, well-known form. Indeed, if all infections with *E. histolytica* caused amebic dysentery, laboratory diagnosis would perhaps be much simpler than it is today. When a microscopist is given a bloody, watery, or mucoid stool

*Presented as part of a *Symposium on Amebiasis* sponsored by The Tropical Disease Center, St. Clare's Hospital, New York, N. Y., and The Merck Company Foundation, Rahway, N. J., held at the Center, September 12, 1970.

he can usually make a direct wet mount in physiological saline and find the organisms, which move in a unidirectional manner and are often filled with ingested red blood cells. Under such conditions there are few problems in identification.

In many cases, a clinical diagnostician can combine good microscopy of the stool with the ability to aspirate or scrape material from ulcers visualized through a sigmoidoscope to make a direct wet mount of these scrapings, and to determine the presence of motile organisms. With skill the diagnostician can fix and stain these organisms in their natural state so that the classical *E. histolytica* with ingested red blood cells is preserved. However, even at this stage of laboratory diagnosis, the ameba must possess a variety of criteria before it is identified as a classic organism. Some researchers have postulated that the term *E. histolytica* should be applied only to those organisms in which ingested red blood cells are seen; in this way microscopic confirmation that the organism is ingesting red blood cells as it invades the tissue would be available. Some misguided workers have developed stricter criteria, and they have postulated that at least two ingested red blood cells should be seen before the organism is called *E. histolytica!*

Although it is true that in these classic cases of amebic dysentery, examination of the bloody stool or aspiration of ulcers of the colon make diagnosis simple, the fact remains that not all infections are classic presentations, and etiologic diagnosis of amebiasis can be difficult and sometimes a frustrating endeavor.

The eventual identification of *E. histolytica* in a stool specimen depends upon organisms being seen under the microscope, generally at high magnification, subjectively fulfilling certain "objective" criteria. These criteria are unique for amebiasis only as much as classic parasitologic diagnosis is unique. Material obtained on a finger cot or during a rectal swab examination is not for the parasitology microscopist. For enteric bacteriology, a tiny bit of feces or rectal swab inoculated into selected media may provide the diagnostician with all the objective information he needs. However, in amebiasis it has long been recommended that some information about the character of the stool specimen be available to the laboratory. Therefore it is generally recommended that a substantial portion of the entire stool be sent to the laboratory so that the microscopist can select the part of the specimen with which to work. In some cases of amebiasis the stool is of the

151

Table I. SUBSTANCES THAT INTERFERE WITH PARASITOLOGIC
EXAMINATION OF FECES

| | |
|---|---|
| *Antidiarrheal preparations*<br>Bismuth, kaolin | *Antacids, Laxatives*<br>Oils, magnesium hydroxide |
| *Radiographic procedures*<br>Barium sulfate | *Enemas*<br>Water, soap solution,<br>irritants, hypertonic<br>salt solutions |
| *Biologically active drugs*<br>Sulfonamides, antibiotic agents,<br>antiprotozoal drugs,<br>anthelmintic agents | |

Adapted from Juniper, 1969[22]

classic diarrhetic or mucoid, bloody type; in other cases formed stools may occur without any blood or evidence that the integrity of the intestinal wall has been impaired. The parasitology laboratory must often decide which type of examination should be performed; this depends on the character of the stool rather than on the patient's symptoms.

A factor in the diagnosis of amebiasis which has become more important in recent years is the knowledge that the examining laboratory should receive a specimen of stool in which there is a reasonable chance that organisms are present. In these days of ready access to antibiotics and other preparations, it is often possible that the patient may have taken "interfering substances" at variable periods before the specimen is submitted to the laboratory. Because of extensive travel to various parts of the world, especially to those considered endemic for amebiasis, it has been recommended that the physician, in obtaining a history from the patient, include Maegraith's question, *"unde venis?"*[21] ("Where have you been?").

It is perhaps also appropriate, considering the possibility of interfering substances in amebiasis, that the physician ask: *"Quibus medicamentes uteris?"* (" What medications or drugs are you now taking?")

Table I, from a recent article by Juniper,[23] lists some of the substances which make it difficut to find organisms in a fecal specimen. The substances reduce the organisms to very low numbers or temporarily eliminate them, so that diagnostic procedures become literally a waste of time. The physician's knowledge of whether or not such substances have been ingested by the patient is invaluable. I know of instances in which numerous stool specimens have been examined over long periods of time while the patients have been taking broad-spectrum antibiotics.

Given the possibility that interfering substances have not been administered to the patient, there are certain guidelines that a microscopist can follow grossly in judging whether or not a particular stool specimen has the characteristics of amebiasis rather than, for example, those of bacillary dysentery. The macroscopical differences between stools in amebiasis and bacillary dysentery have been well outlined recently by Stamm.[23]

Such guidelines for gross distinctions should perhaps be used only by experienced observers. The tendency of the inexperienced might be to make a specific diagnosis of the stool macroscopically, that is, by its solid or liquid state. whether or not it was streaked with blood, whether fecal elements were present, and whether the odor was offensive or alkaline. In amebiasis such "long distance diagnosis" without resort to microscopy is not to be encouraged.

The direct wet mount of a stool, in physiological saline, has always been the standby for initial examination. The procedure for making a direct wet mount is simple. A bit of stool is placed on a slide and emulsified in the saline; a coverslip is added, and a search is made of the entire preparation for trophic or cystic forms. The consistency of the preparation should be such that newsprint can easily be read through it.

In those instances in which the stools are watery, loose, or soft, and rapid passage through the colon has perhaps taken place, there is a tendency for trophic forms of the organism to predominate. A bit of Nair's solution[24] added to the wet mount aids in delineating the morphology of the trophic amebas. In a more solid specimen, if it is produced in chronic amebiasis during such times as the intervals between attacks of diarrhea or dysentery, the stools contain more cystic forms. In such cases the usual procedure is to make a wet mount in physiological saline and also a preparation containing a bit of Dobell's iodine, which helps delineate the glycogen mass, nuclear elements, and the chromatoid bodies, if these are present. For many years some workers have added 0.5% eosin to the physiological saline solution. In this preparation the living cysts, which do not take up the eosin, stand out as refractile bodies and can be detected easily. After this comes the difficult part in diagnosis. Organisms that are seen must be distinguished by species, that is, they must be classified as *Entamoeba histolytica*, *E. hartmanni*, *E. coli*, *Endolimax nana*, *Iodamoeba butschlii*, or perhaps as a mixture of many species, as sometimes occurs.[25, 29]

The number of stools which should be examined before infection with *E. histolytica* is ruled out has been the subject of several reports.[11, 26] The rule accepted by many workers is that not less than three normally passed specimens obtained over a period of 7 to 10 days should be examined to determine whether organisms are present. This is the standard "O & P times 3" which appears on so many laboratory forms. The percentage of infections which are detected, based on the number of stools examined, has been reported on by Svensson[26] and by Stamm.[11]

Quoting several sources, Stamm stated that the consensus was that about 30% of the positives present would be found by a single examination. Estimates are that 75 to 95% of the infections are found after examination of the third specimen. How many specimens a laboratory should examine after the third one depends as much on the physician as on the laboratory. Continued stool examinations may occasionally be fruitful. However, there is always the danger that the pressure to find *E. histolytica* may persuade a microscopist that what he thought were artifacts were actually the elusive sarcodine. Strange as it may seem, one occasionally hears the statement: "The patient has amebiasis; therefore, there should be *E. histolytica* in his stool specimen."

Cathartics such as buffered phosphosoda are used to obtain "purged" specimens and are sometimes recommended[7, 9, 13, 15, 22] to increase the yield of organisms in stools. The value of using three normally passed stools as well as purged specimens was noted by Sawitz.[27] Reports by Yarinsky and Sternberg[28] list good reasons for examining always both the first and second specimens taken after a purge.

A stool of recent passage, an experienced microscopist, and time enough for examination are three conditions that rarely coexist. Indeed, in many laboratories, parasitological examinations of feces sometimes occupy a relatively small period of the time of a technologist who is obliged to function also as a bacteriologist, serologist, or hematologist. Separate parasitological laboratories exist in relatively few institutions, such as large hospitals, state health departments, or federal establishments. If an examination of a fresh stool can be accomplished by a skilled microscopist within a period of one to two hours it is one of the best and most valuable types of examination and is not to be discredited.

The situation in which the corner of a laboratory contains stool cartons collected throughout the day and awaiting examination is not unusual in some institutions. Many years ago it was thought that the amebas coming out in the stool specimen from a warm body should continue to be kept as warm as possible. It was then customary to place stools in a 37° C. incubator if there was to be a long delay in examination. However, it is now recommended that a stool be kept at room temperature or even at 4° C. in a refrigerator both for aesthetic reasons and also in order to retard the action of bacteria which may destroy trophic forms. Experience has shown, however, that a stool specimen may be passed hours before it is examined for parasites. To obviate the problems that arise during the interval between passage and examination, and because of the difficulty in finding sparse organisms, a number of techniques, ancillary to the direct wet mount examination, have been developed. Solutions are now used to preserve the specimen so that it can be examined at leisure, and procedures are used for concentrating the organisms in a small amount of material.

It is interesting that many of the standard procedures in use today for the diagnosis of amebiasis were developed 15 to 30 years ago. In some fecal specimens amebas may be so few that many normal specimens or even purged stools must be examined before the culprit is found. For years it was thought that if the organisms could be concentrated in a small amount of material it would be advantageous. The time spent searching through slide after slide would be eliminated. A technique which concentrates trophic forms of ameba in loose, soft, or watery specimens has not yet been developed.

One of the first laboratory techniques developed for concentrating parasitic organisms in stools was the zinc-sulfate procedure of Faust and his co-workers.[30] Floating the protozoan cysts, helminth eggs, and other portions of the feces in a solution of 33% zinc sulfate, at a specific gravity of about 1.18 to 1.2, enabled the microscopist to "corral" many organisms in a small amount of fluid. This is a very useful procedure. Trophozoites, if not destroyed, are generally distorted, sometimes beyond recognition. The zinc-sulfate concentrating technique, still widely used, was developed in 1938.

In 1948 Ritchie[31] introduced the formalin ether (FE) concentration technique, which has been modified slightly by some workers.[32] It is also a procedure used in general parasitologic diagnosis, that is, for the recovery of helminth larvae and eggs as well as protozoan cysts. Ritchie's FE procedure uses a very common ingredient of the laboratory—the pathologist's "*aqua eterna*," formaldehyde. The stool specimen is placed in a tube containing formalin, a small amount of ether is added, and then the tube is centrifuged. The individual protozoan cysts, helminth larvae, and eggs are separated from most of the fecal debris and can be detected in the sediment.

The FE technique of Ritchie is widely used in a variety of laboratories. It is especially useful because it can be performed with no loss of morphologic integrity in specimens which have been previously collected and preserved in 5 to 10% formalin. However, the FE technique does not concentrate the trophic forms to any degree and is not well suited for the concentration of cysts of *Giardia lamblia*.

The Army's contribution to parasitologic diagnosis in the late 1940's was Ritchie's FE technique; this was followed quickly by the Navy's contribution in 1953, when Sapero and Lawless[33] introduced the merthiolate-iodine formalin (MIF) procedure. This was another method of treating fecal specimens that assured the preservation of any organisms present; also identification could be performed at leisure. The merthiolate and iodine provided a polychromatic staining of the protozoan nuclei, chromatoid bars, glycogen masses, and cell membranes. Both the MIF and FE procedures can be used for specimens collected far away, both in distance and time, from a central diagnostic laboratory.

A highly significant contribution to diagnostic parasitology was made by the Public Health Service when the polyvinyl alcohol (PVA) fixative technique was developed by Brooke and Goldman.[34] With the PVA fixative, it was possible to collect stool specimens and to preserve the fragile trophic forms so that their integrity was maintained and distinct morphological characters (nuclear beading, cytoplasm, cell membrane) were preserved for subsequent staining and critical observation.

The PVA fixative only preserves the organisms, which must be stained before the morphology can be critically evaluated. Few routine diagnostic laboratories today use the long Heidenhain iron-hematoxylin

156

## USE OF PVA-FIXATIVE TECHNIQUE
## FOR SUBMITTING STOOL SPECIMENS TO BE EXAMINED FOR PARASITES
### ADAPTED FROM BROOKE AND GOLDMAN, 1949

NOTE: BOTH SOFT AND FORMED SPECIMENS SHOULD BE SUBMITTED BY THIS METHOD. SPECIMENS MUST BE FRESH WHEN PLACED IN VIALS.

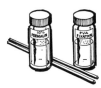

**1** The kit consists of two glass vials (one with 10% formalin, and one with PVA).

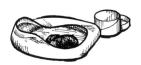

**2** The stool should be passed into a dry container. Urine should not be passed into the same container.

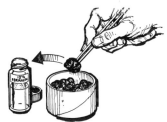

**3** Using applicator sticks, place a quantity of the stool into the 10% formalin (ratio of 5 parts formalin to 1 stool).

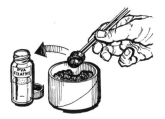

**4** Place a similar quantity into the vial containing the PVA fixative.

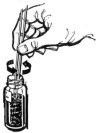

**5** Thoroughly break up specimen in the 10% formalin and PVA fixative. Shake vigorously.

**6** Place the two vials so as to protect against breakage. Enclose appropriate identification and mail or deliver to laboratory.

DHEW, PHS, HSM, NCDC

ATLANTA, GA. — JUNE 1969

techniques since it is time-consuming and subject to errors in the processes of destaining and mordanting. However, when critical examination of protozoan morphology is needed, it is still useful and largely unsurpassed.

For routine diagnostic purposes, the trichrome stain of Wheatley,[35] developed in 1951, is useful since it affords critical staining and presents a pleasant polychromatic picture. The short iron-hematoxylin procedure of Tompkins and Miller[36] is favored by some workers; like the Wheatley trichrome, it can be used with stool specimens that have been preserved by means of PVA. Many workers advocate the formalin-PVA preservation method seen in the accompanying plate for the complete examination of a stool for all parasites, including amebas. This method can be used for routine office, clinic, or hospital work as well as during surveys or on those occasions in which several hours or even days may elapse between collection and examination.

Although diagnostic techniques for amebiasis in particular and parasites in general were developed many years ago there are a number of useful newer procedures which need only be evaluated by various workers over a period of time for more widespread acceptance. Burrows[37] recently reported a much needed improvement in the method of preparing PVA-fixative, and he introduced in 1967[38] an additional fixative, the "PAF," for preservation of diagnostic stages of protozoa and helminths. Arensburger and Markell[39] developed a useful combination direct-concentrate procedure in 1962, and Silva in 1969[40] reported the efficacy of a "larvoocyst" apparatus which utilizes zinc sulfate flotation to collect larvae, eggs, and protozoan cysts.

In 1966[41] Mitchell reported that the penetration of mordant and hematoxylin was improved by the addition of dimethyl sulfoxide to the solutions. In the same year Alger[42] described a modification of the trichrome stain which was simple, precise, and rapid, and could be used by inexperienced workers. A few years ago, in our own laboratory, we investigated[43] the chlorazol-black combination fixative-stain developed by Kohn in 1960,[44] and we found that it was very useful, especially for small laboratories or clinics which do not examine large numbers of stools and do not have the various solutions, stains, and equipment necessary for diagnosis.

The use of cultures for the detection of *E. histolytica* in stool specimens has a long history. The LER medium of Boeck and Drbohlav[45] developed in 1925 is still used today, as are the liver extract medium of Cleveland and Collier,[46] the egg infusion of Balamuth,[47] and the alcohol-egg extract of Nelson.[48] Generally the culturing of stools for intestinal amebas is carried out in laboratories in which parasitologic diagnosis is an ongoing activity, not a sideline. Some workers have minimized the use of cultures for routine diagnosis. None of the culture techniques allow the growth and multiplication of *E. histolytica* alone; therefore if cultures are positive and organisms are seen, the microscopist is still faced with the problem of differentiating *E. histoytica* from other amebas in the media.

The experience of some diagnosticians, however, indicates that the use of cultures, in addition to the other diagnostic methods in amebiasis, can be valuable. The recent positive results of McQuay,[49] who used his charcoal medium[50] for cultivating the stools of furloughed missionaries in Chicago, and the positive results of Robinson,[18] who used his newly developed culture medium in Greenwich, England, speak well for the use of cultures as a part of the armamentarium of techniques for the diagnosis of amebiasis.

Although diagnosing amebic infections of the intestine probably constitutes most of the work of the routine laboratory, some strains of *E. histolytica* are capable of penetrating and thriving in tissues other than the wall of the colon. The gynecologist, for example, may encounter diagnostic problems in amebiasis; these were recently pointed out by Munguia et al.[51] in their detection of *E. histolytica* in Papanicolaou smears.

The etiologic diagnosis of extraintestinal amebiasis is difficult. Recovery of organisms from tissues such as the liver, the primary focus of the amebas outside the intestine, is not very successful in many diagnostic laboratories. The average laboratory is generally not called upon to search for or identify amebas in tissues from liver biopsy or so called amebic hepatitis.

Fluid obtained from a liver abscess by open drainage or closed aspiration is generally the material which the laboratory receives for examination. Such fluid may be of the "typical" anchovy-paste color and consistency, and a positive diagnosis of amebiasis is often concluded on the recovery of such typical fluid without demonstration of the organism. However, as pointed out by Wilmot,[52] fluid from an amebic liver abscess may be white, cream-colored, greenish, or yellowish. Foul-smelling, greenish or yellowish fluid indicative of bacterial infection does not rule out the fact that the fluid may have originally been sterile. Maddison et al.[53] pointed out that the sterility of the abscess fluid may be proportional to the number of times aspiration has been attemped.

Just as the laboratory can seldom find amebas in stool specimens if the patient is taking interfering substances, the chances are likewise small that isolation and identification of organisms will be successful if the pus from a liver abscess cannot be expected to contain organisms. This is usually the case when the first portions of the fluid drained or aspirated from an abscess are sent to the laboratory. Some authors[12, 54] have pointed out that amebas are found at the periphery of the abscess and are more abundant in the last part of the aspirate or drainage recovered. Such fluid shows the typical red color. With the removal of the static fluid pressure, the wall of the abscess shrinks or collapses, expressing amebas and blood from the tissue.

Lello[54] several years ago outlined a procedure employing streptodornase and streptokinase to free the amebas from the thick coagulum of pus which is often obtained in drainage from liver abscesses. The resultant fluid can be either examined as a wet mount preparation, fixed to slides, placed in PVA for staining, or inoculated into the standard culture media already mentioned. Culture media inoculated with fluid from a liver abscess must also be inoculated or "seeded" with bacteria, particularly if the aspirate fluid is sterile, since amebas seem to thrive better *in vitro* with bacteria. Inoculating abscess fluid into a highly specialized medium such as the axenic type developed by Diamond[55] may be useful but is not recommended as a routine procedure. Mixed bacterial flora or monoconcomitants such as *Escherichia coli* or *Clostridium welchii*[56] are often used with the initiation and maintenance of cultures of amebas.

The number of successful isolations of *E. histolytica* from extraintestinal sites are very few compared with isolations from intestinal infections. Clinical impression, history, and response to chemotherapy are often the only choices open to the physician because of difficulties in obtaining an etiologic diagnosis. Serologic study has been resorted to as an aid in cases in which the organism is difficult to find.

Many years ago serologic techniques were used in the diagnosis of amebiasis, both for intestinal and extraintestinal disease. Difficulties in obtaining standardized antigens, the problem of serologically false nega-

Table II. RESULTS OF RECENT SEROLOGIC TESTS FOR AMEBIASIS

| Serologic test | Amebic Liver abscess No. sera | Amebic Liver abscess % Positive | Symptomatic intestinal amebiasis No. sera | Symptomatic intestinal amebiasis % Positive | Author | Year |
|---|---|---|---|---|---|---|
| IHA* | 35 | 100% | 133 | 98% | Kessel et al. | 1965 |
| IHA | 121 | 96% | 83 | 82% | Milgram et al. | 1966 |
| IHA | | | 63 | 85% | Healy | 1968 |
| IHA | 31 | 87% | 168 | 81% | Krupp | 1970 |
| IHA | 16 | 75% | 6 | 100% | Prakash et al. | 1970 |
| IHA | 16 | 87% | 20 | 85% | Halpern et al. | 1967 |
| IHA | 48 | 100% | 41 | 90% | Thompson et al. | 1968 |
| IHA | 47 | 92% | | | Savant and Chaicumpa | 1969 |
| CF† | 20 | 100% | 92 | 90% | Kessel et al. | 1965 |
| CF | 55 | 100% | | | Kasliwal et al. | 1966 |
| CF | 31 | 84% | 30 | 63% | Thompson et al. | 1968 |
| IFA‡ | 18 | 100% | 10 | 80% | Coudert et al. | 1968 |
| IFA | 61 | 95% | 40 | 75% | Jeanes | 1969 |
| IFA | 33 | 91% | 33 | 75% | Boonpucknavig and Nairn | 1967 |
| IFA | 42 | 100% | 23 | 91% | Ambroise-Thomas et al. | 1969 |
| SAFA§ | 15 | 100% | 12 | 100% | Gore and Sadun | 1968 |
| IFA | 22 | 90% | 32 | 84% | Goldman | 1966 |
| Gel diffusion | 528 | 94% | | | Powell et al. | 1965 |
| Gel diffusion | | | 400 | 92% | Powell et al. | 1967 |
| Gel diffusion | 33 | 93% | 32 | 66% | Boonpucknavig and Nairn | 1967 |
| Gel diffusion | 12 | 92% | 22 | 95% | Halpern et al. | 1967 |
| Gel diffusion | 49 | 80% | 41 | 54% | Thompson et al. | 1968 |
| Tube precipitin | 150 | 97% | 150 | 89% | Powell | 1968 |
| Immunoelectrophoresis | 93 | 97% | 6 | 67% | Savant and Chaicumpa | 1969 |
| Bentonite flocculation | 90 | 93% | 50 | 86% | Tupasi and Healy | 1970 |
| Latex agglutination | 100 | 98% | 100 | 96% | Morris et al. | 1970 |
| Bentonite phagocytosis | 17 | 100% | 24 | 96% | Halpern et al. | 1967 |

*Indirect hemagglutination test
†Complement fixation test

‡Indirect fluorescent antibody test
§Soluble antigen fluorescent antibody test

tive and false positive reactions, and the problem of ameba-bacteria antigenic complexes limited the use of serology in diagnosis. In the past decade, however, there has been a renewed interest in the judicious use of serologic techniques, particularly for amebic liver abscess.

This interest has been stimulated to some extent by the advances in the field of serology in general, partly by the development of more sophisticated techniques for making purer antigens and partly by the knowledge that in extraintestinal amebiasis, classic isolation techniques are difficult and often unrewarding.

The results obtained by several groups of workers over the past decade who employed serologic techniques for the detection of amebic infections may be seen in Table II. The list is not exhaustive, since many workers published preliminary papers prior to the reference cited. Virtually every type of serologic procedure has been employed for both symptomatic intestinal and extraintestinal amebiasis. Various workers have obtained different results. The difference in positivity rates reflects not only differences in the populations studied but also individual variations in the criteria used to determine positive and negative serologic results. The number of references in Table II, however, indicates that a sizeable body of literature[57-76] now exists, attesting to the use of serologic techniques. The list continues to grow. For the perplexing problem of suspected amebic liver abscess, in particular, serology would seem to be very promising as a useful diagnostic tool.

In summarizing this review I am encouraged by the progress which has been made. Time-tested, reliable techniques are still in use. Periodically the literature is nourished by the publication of a new technique or a modification of an older method; the new data help to sharpen the tests for this protozoan parasite, so important in medicine and public health. Serology has a place in the laboratory diagnosis of amebiasis. The limits of serologic diagnosis in intestinal amebiasis have been pointed out by some,[66] and doubtless there will be other critical evaluations.

A prospective appraisal of the diagnosis of amebiasis is not within the purview of this presentation. Nearly 20 years ago a group of 93 qualified workers examined the subject in some depth.[10] Results did not show universal agreement on the criteria for diagnosis. Perhaps it is time for another analysis.

If I were asked to forecast the future of laboratory diagnosis, I should say that the outlook is good. The increasing role of serology was noted above. For classic etiologic diagnosis, the passage of the Clinical Laboratories Improvement Act of 1967[77] has stimulated the use of referee laboratories, reference or check specimens, plus the inclusion of quality-control methods in the laboratory diagnosis of all parasitic diseases. Private and governmental institutions are now using evaluation specimens to upgrade and check diagnostic proficiency. Preliminary analysis and results of laboratory proficiency indicate that such evaluations are needed, but the future does look bright.

## REFERENCES

1. Burrows, R. B.,: *Microscopical Diagnosis of the Parasites of Man.* New Haven, Yale Univ. Press, 1965.
2. Markell, E. K. and Voge, M.: *Diagnostic Medical Parasitology.* Philadelphia, Saunders, 1965.
3. Melvin, D. M. and Brooke, M. M.: *Laboratory Procedures for the Diagnosis of Intestinal Parasites.* Public Health Service Bulletin No. 1969, 1969, pp. IX, 166.
4. Spencer, F. M. and Monroe, L. S.: *The Color Atlas of Intestinal Parasites.* Springfield, Thomas, 1961.
5. Anderson, H. H., Bostick, W. L. and Johnstone, H. G.: *Amebiasis, Pathology, Diagnosis, and Chemotherapy.* Springfield, Thomas, 1953.
6. Faust, E. C.: *Amebiasis.* Springfield, Thomas, 1954.
7. Brooke, M. M.: *Amebiasis: Methods in Laboratory Diagnosis.* Atlanta, Comm. Dis. Center, 1958.
8. U.S. Public Health Service: *Amebiasis: Laboratory Diagnosis Part I, Life Cycle of Entamobea histolytica. Part II, Identfication of Intestinal Amebae. Part III, Laboratory Procedures.* Public Health Service Pub. No. 1187, 1964.
9. Swartzwelder, C.: Laboratory dignosis of amebiasis. *Amer. J. Clin. Path. 22:* 379-95, 1952.
10. Brooke, M. M., Otto, G., Brady, F., Faust, E. C., Mackie, T. F. and Most, H.: An analysis of a memorandum on the diagnosis of amebiasis. *Amer J. Trop. Med. 2:*593-612, 1953.
11. Stamm, W. P.: The diagnosis of Clinical amoebiasis. *Trans. Roy. Soc. Trop. Med. Hyg. 51:*306-12, 1957.
12. Brooke, M. M.: Laboratory diagnosis of amebiasis. *Proc. VI Int. Congr. Trop, Med. Mal. 3:*369-84, 1958.
13. Brooke, M. M.: Laboratory regimens for diagnosis of intestinal amebiasis by gastroenterologists. *Proc. World. Congr. Gastroent.,* pp. 754-58, 1958.
14. Healy, G. R.: The laboratory diagnosis of amebiasis. *Amer. J. Gastroent. 42:* 191-97, 1964.
15. Goldman, M.: Identification and diagnosis of *Entamoeba histolytica. Amer. J. Gastroent. 41:* 362-65, 1964.
16. Wright, R.: Amoebiasis—A diagnostic problem in Great Britain. *Brit. Med. J. 1:*957-59, 1966.
17. Prakash, O. and Tandon, B. N.: Intestinal parasites with special reference to *Entamoeba histolytica* complex as revealed by routine, concentration and cultural examination of stool specimens from gastro-intestinal symptoms. *Indian J. Med. Res. 54:*1-5, 1966.
18. Robinson, G. L.: The laboratory diagnosis of human parasitic amoebae. *Trans. Roy. Soc. Trop. Med. Hyg. 62:* 285-94, 1968.
19. Elsdon-Dew, R.: Amoebiasis: Its meaning and diagnosis. *South Afr. Med. J.* 43:483-86, 1969.
20. Faust, E. C.: The multiple facets of *Entamoeba histolytica* infection. *Int. Rev. Trop. Med. 1:*43-76, 1960.
21. Maegraith, B.: *Unde Venis? Lancet,* Feb. 23:401-04, 1963.
22. Juniper, K.: Parasitic Diseases of the Intestinal Tract. In: *Gastroenterologic Medicine.* Paulson, M., ed. 1969, pp. 472-560.
23. Stamm, W. P.: Laboratory aids in the management of some common diarrhoeas in the tropics. *Trans. Roy. Soc. Trop. Med. Hyg. 59:*712-15, 1965.
24. Nair, E. P.: Rapid staining of intestinal amoebae in wet mounts. *Nature 172:* 1051, 1953.
25. Healy, G. R., Gleason, N. N., Bokat, R., Pond, H. and Roper, M.: Prevalence of ascariasis and amebiasis in Cherokee Indian school children. *Public Health Rep. 84:*907-14, 1969.
26. Svensson, R.: Studies on human intestinal protozoa. *Acta Medica Scandinavica,* Suppl. LXX, pp. 1-115, 1935.
27. Sawitz, W. C.: *Medical Parasitology for Medical Students and Practicing Physicians.* New York, McGraw-Hill, 1956.
28. Yarinsky, A. E. and Sternberg, S. deB.: A study of paired, purged stool specimens for the recovery of *Entamoeba histolytica. Amer. J. Clin. Path. 40:* 598-600, 1963.

29. Elsdon-Dew, R.: The epidemiology of amoebiasis. *Advances Parasit. 6*:1-62, 1968.

30. Faust, E. C., D'Antoni, J. S., Odum, V., Miller, M. J., Peres, C., Sawitz, W., Thomen, L.F., Tobie, J. and Walker, J. H.: Critical study of clinical laboratory technics for diagnosis of protozoan cysts and helminth eggs in feces. *Amer. J. Trop. Med. 18*:169-83, 1938.

31. Ritchie, L. S.: An ether sedimentation technique for routine stool examinations. *Bull. U.S. Army Med. Dept. 8*:326, 1956.

32. Ridley, D. S. and Hawgood, B. C.: The value of formol-ether concentration of faecal cysts and ova. *J. Clin. Path. 9*:74-76, 1956.

33. Sapero, J. J. and Lawless, D. K.: The "MIF" stain-preservation technique for the identification of intestinal protozoa. *Amer. J. Trop. Med. 2*:613-19, 1953.

34. Brooke, M. M. and Goldman, M.: Polyvinyl alcohol-fixative as a preservative and adhesive for protozoa in dysenteric stools and other liquid material. *J. Lab. Clin. Med. 34*:1554-60, 1949.

35. Wheatley, W. B.: A rapid staining procedure for intestinal amoebae and flagellates. *Amer. J. Clin. Path. 21*: 990-91, 1951.

36. Tompkins, V. N. and Miller, J. K.: Staining intestinal protozoa with iron-hematoxylin-phosphotungstic acid. *Amer. J. Clin. Path. 17*:755-57, 1947.

37. Burrows, R. B.: Improved preparation of polyvinyl alcohol-HgCl₂ fixative used for fecal smears. *Stain Technol. 42*: 93-95, 1967.

38. Burrows, R. B.: A new fixative and technics for the diagnosis of intestinal parasites. *Amer. J. Clin. Path. 48*: 342-46, 1967.

39. Arensburger, K. E. and Markell, E. K.: A simple combination direct smear and fecal concentration for permanent stained preparations. *Amer. J. Clin. Path. 34*:50-51, 1960.

40. Silva, M.: An ultra-rapid appartus for diagnosing intestinal parasitoses: A larvoocyst detector. *Bull. WHO 41*: 962-64, 1969.

41. Mitchell, H.: A simple method of permanent staining of intestinal parasites, using dimethyl sulfoxide. *Techn. Bull. Regist. Med. Techn. 36*:45-46, 1966.

42. Alger, N.: A simple, rapid, precise stain for intestinal protozoa. *Amer. J. Clin. Path. 45*:361-62, 1968.

43. Gleason, N. N. and Healy, G. R.: Modification and evaluation of Kohn's one-step staining technique for intestinal protozoa in feces or tissue. *Amer. J. Clin. Path. 43*:494-96, 1965.

44. Kohn, J.: A one-stage permanent staining method for faecal protozoa. *Dapim. Refuiim.* (Tel-Aviv) *19*:160-61, 1960.

45. Boeck, W. C. and Drbohlav, J.: The cultivation of *Entamoeba histolytica. Amer. J. Hyg. 5*:371 407, 1925.

46. Cleveland, L. R. and Collier, J.: The various improvements in the cultivation of *Entamoeba histolytica. Amer. J. Hyg. 12*:606-13, 1930.

47. Balamuth, W.: Improved egg yolk infusion for cultivation of *Endamoeba histolytica* and other intestinal protozoa. *Amer. J. Clin. Path. 16*:380, 1946.

48. Nelson, E. C.: Alcoholic extract medium for the diagnosis and cultivation of *Endamoeba histolytica. Amer. J. Trop. Med. 27*:525, 1947.

49. McQuay, R.: Parasitologic studies in a group of furloughed missionaries. I. Intestinal protozoa. *Amer. J. Trop. Med. Hyg. 16*:154-60, 1967.

50. McQuay, R. M.: Charcoal medium for growth and maintenance of large and small races of *Entamoeba histolytica. Amer. J. Clin. Path. 26*:1137-41, 1956.

51. Munguia, H., Franco, E. and Valenzuela, P.: Diagnosis of genital amebiasis in women by the standard Papanicolaou technique. *Amer. J. Obstet. Gynec. 94*: 181-88, 1966.

52. Wilmot, A. J.: *Clinical Amoebiasis.* Philadelphis, Davis, 1962.

53. Maddison, S. E., Powell, S. J. and Elsdon-Dew, R.: Bacterial infection of amoebic liver abscess. *Med. Proc. 5*: 514-15, 1959.

54. Lello, M. A.: A method for the examination of hepatic abscess for *Entamoeba histolytica. Lab. News & Views. 3*:2,1954.

55. Diamond, L.: Techniques of axenic cultivation of *Entamoeba hitolytica* Schau-

dinn, 1903 and *E. histolytica*-like amebae. *J. Parasit. 54*:1047-56, 1968.

56. Freedman, L., Maddison, S. E. and Elsdon-Dew, R.: Monoxenic cultures of *Entamoeba histolytica* derived from human liver abscess. *S. Afr. J. Med. Sci. 23*:9-10, 1958.

57. Kessel, J. F., Lewis, W. P., Molina-Pasquel, C. and Turner, J. A.: Indirect hemagglutination and complement fixation tests in amebiasis. *Amer. J. Trop. Med. 14*:540-51, 1965.

58. Powell, S. J., Maddison, S. E., Wilmot, A. J. and Elsdon-Dew, R.: Amoebic gel diffusion precipitin test. Clinical evaluation in amoebic liver abscess. *Lancet 2*:602-03, 1965.

59. Milgram, E. A., Healy, G. R. and Kagan, I. G.: Studies on the use of the indirect hemagglutination test in the diagnosis of amebiasis *Gastroenterology 50*:645-49, 1966.

60. Kasliwal, R. M., Kenney, M. Gupta, M. L., Sethi, J. P., Tatz, J. S. and Illes, C. H.: Signficance of the complement-fixation test in diagnosis of amebiasis in an endemic area. *Brit. Med. J. 1*:837-38, 1966.

61. Powell, S. J., Maddison, S. E., Hodgson, R. G. and Elsdon-Dew, R.: Amoebic gel diffusion precipitin test. Clinical evaluation in acute amoebic dysentery. *Lancet 1*:566-67, 1966.

62. Boonpucknavig, S. and Nairn, R. C.: Serological diagnosis of amebiasis by immunofluorescence. *J. Clin. Path. 20*: 875-78, 1967.

63. Halpern, B., Young, J. J., Dolkart, J., Armour, P. D., III and Dolkart, R. E.: The serologic response of patients with amebiasis compared by gel diffusion, hemagglutination, and phagocytosis techniques with a common *Entamoeba histolytica* antigen preparation. *J. Lab. Clin. Med. 69*:467-71, 1967.

64. Goldman, M.: Evaluation of a fluorescent antibody test for amebiasis using two widely differing ameba strains as antigen. *Amer. J. Trop. Med. 15*:694-700, 1966.

65. Thompson, P. E., Graedel, S. K., Schneider, C. R., Stucki, W. P. and Gordon, R.: Preparation and evaluation of standarized amoeba antigen from

axenic cultures of *Entamoeba histolytica. Bull. WHO 39*:349-65, 1968.

66. Healy, G. R.: The use of and limitations to the indirect hemagglutination test in the diagnosis of intestinal amebiasis. *Health Lab. Sci. 5*:174-79, 1968.

67. Gore, R. W. and Sadun, E. H.: Soluble antigen fluorescent antibody test for amebiasis *Exp. Parasit 22*:316-20, 1968.

68. Coudert, J., Garin, J. P., Ambroise-Thomas, P. and Georget, J. P.: Diagnostic serologique de l'amebiasis par immuno-fluorescence. Resultats de 160 examens. *Bull. Soc. Path. Exot. 60*: 44-52, 1967.

69. Powell, S. J.: The capillary tube precipitin test. A rapid serologic aid to clinical diagnosis in invasive amebiasis. *Amer. J. Trop. Med. 17*:840-43, 1968.

70. Savant, T. and Chaicumpa, W.: Immun oelectrophoresis test for amebiasis. *Bull. WHO 40*:343-53, 1969.

71. Ambroise-Thomas, P. and Truong, T. K.: Le diagnostic serologique de l' ambiase humaine par la technique des anticorps fluorescents. *Bull. WHO. 40*: 103-12, 1969.

72. Jeanes, C. L.: Evaluation in clincal practice of the fluorescent amoebic antibody test. *J. Clin. Path. 22*:427-29, 1969.

73. Krupp, I.: Antibody response in intestinal and extraintestinal amebiasis. *Amer. J. Trop. Med. 19*:57-62, 1970.

74. Prakash, O., Tandon, B. N., Bhalla, I., Ray, A. K. and Vinayak, V. K.: In direct hemagglutination and ameba-immobilization tests and their evaluation in intestinal and extraintestinal amebiasis. *Amer. J. Trop. Med. 18*: 670-75, 1969.

75. Tupasi, T. E. and Healy, G. R.: Adaptation of the Bozicevich trichinella bentonite flocculation test for the diagnosis of amebiasis. *Amer. J. Trop. Med. 19*: 43-48, 1970.

76. Morris, M. N., Powell, S. J. and Elsdon-Dew, R.: Latex agglutination test for invasive amebiasis. *Lancet, June* 27: 1362-63, 1970.

77. Clinical Laboratories Improvement Act of 1967. Notice of Effective Date. *Fed. Reg. 33*:15297-303, 1968.

165

# SYMPOSIUM ON AMEBIASIS*

## Panel Discussion

# THE SEROLOGY OF AMEBIASIS

GEORGE R. HEALY, Ph.D. AND KEVIN M. CAHILL, M.D., *editors*

RONALD ELSDON-DEW, M.D.; KERRISON JUNIPER, JR., M.D.;

S. JOHN POWELL, M.D.

DR. GEORGE HEALY. Serology has a useful place in the diagnosis of amebiasis. We all agree that in cases of liver abscess, serology is very good; in cases of invasive intestinal amebiasis, it is also useful.

When we talk about how good something is we might profitably begin by showing its limitations. I call to your attention a seroepidemiologic study on sera from Cherokee Indian school children in North Carolina (Figure 1). These children had prevalence rates of 50% for *Ascaris lumbricoides* infections, 39% for *Trichuris trichiura* infections, and a variety of intestinal protozoa. In 1965 we found 11% of them infected with *Entamoeba histolytica*. The frequency-distribution curve of the titers suggests that there were probably no cases of invasive amebiasis. This supposition is supported by the low positive serology, a fact corroborated by the experience of the physicians in the Indian Hospital. The point to be noted is that serology and stool positivity do not necessarily have to agree; they may mean different things. Figure 2 demonstrates the converse of this; two populations were examined by stool examinations and serology, with invasive amebiasis confirmed in population B by a high incidence of serologic as well as stool positives. The seroepidemiologic curve extended farther out and had a peak titer of 1:1024, which is consistent with our results in present or recently acquired clinical amebiasis.

As the use of serology in amebiasis becomes more accepted and commercial diagnostic preparations become available to the individual physician within the next year or two, some caution has to be taken in the interpretation of serologic results. In some of the tests used in

---

*Held by The Tropical Disease Center, St. Clare's Hospital, New York, N. Y., and The Merck Company Foundation, Rahway, N. J., at the Center, September 12, 1970.

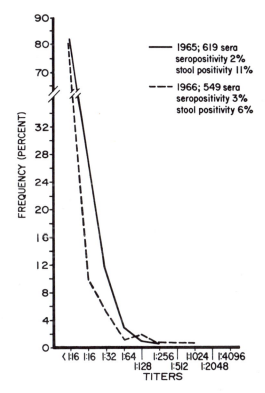

Fig. 1. Frequency distribution of IHA titers to *Entamoeba histolytica* antigen. Cherokee Indian school children. Reproduced by permission from Healy, G. R., Kagan, I. G. and Gleason, N. N. *Health Lab. Sci.* 7:109-16, 1970.

amebiasis serology, the titers drop slowly over a long period of time after chemotherapy. The titer reported on the serum from an individual may be due to an antibody response which was stimulated by experience with the organisms weeks or months prior to the test. The current symptoms in the patient may not be at all related to the serology of amebiasis.

Dr. Elsdon-Dew. We have been studying amebiasis in Durban for a long time. Initially we tried doing complement-fixation tests but our results were just a bit confusing. We obtained very good results in

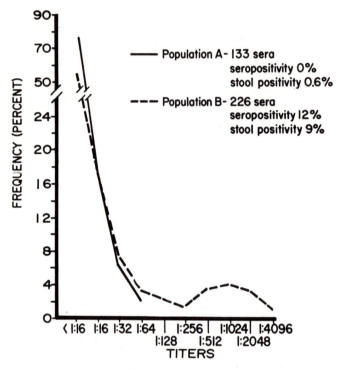

Fig. 2. Frequency distribution of IHA titers to *Entamoeba histolytica* antigen. Calion, Ark. Reproduced by permission from Healy, G. R., Kagan, I. G. and Gleason, N. N. *Health Lab. Sci.* 7:109-16, 1970.

cases of liver abscess (I think there was approximately a 98% positivity of the sera from liver abscesses). We had cases, however, in which we could not find the ameba after careful search and in which there were positive reactions. Sera from cases of amebic dysentery gave us, I think, a bit more than 80% positivity or thereabout. This led us to believe that though there was something useful in serology (we did not know what it was), it was well that we should attempt to do some developmental studies. Complement fixation and indirect hemagglutination (the latter at that time was very much in its youth) were good! Fluorescent antibody tests were not available at that time. I determined, however, that we should use the simplest possible system that would allow us to analyze our results critically. To that end, happily, just at that time the Ouchterlony agar-gel procedure came into use.

This is a very good technique since by means of it one can identify individual antigen-antibody reactions. It was about this time that we started working with Dr. S. John Powell and his clinical group. This association gave us an inestimable advantage in that we could obtain adequately documented cases with which to evaluate our tests. This was fortunate, for a test must be evaluated against some sort of known standard, and we knew the exact clinical history of every case; our number of these cases now exceeds 30,000. To make a long story short, we found that the gel-diffusion test is very good. We interpret our findings in this way: a positive reaction implies present or past invasion with *E. histolytica*. We find that many cyst passers show no detectable antibodies at all. In these cases we assume the amebas have remained in the commensal phase and have not traversed the barrier of the mucosal surface. One may be leading with one's chin in this statement, but I am pretty sure this is correct.

Last year I was able to carry out another study in a mental institution in Holland. We had all the parasitological findings, and we found that a large proportion of cyst passers were serologically negative. When we checked our findings with the clinical histories (here we had patients who were captive and we were able to obtain their complete medical histories) the serology fitted entirely.

So it may be asked: "What is the place of serology in the diagnosis of amebiasis"? I think that in acute amebic dysentery, the microscope is still the tool. This method is fast and it is neat! But there are times when serology is, practically speaking, a little faster, as in liver abscesses. Our physicians in Durban are pretty good at clinical diagnosis but one may come up against a situation in which it is not known whether a palpable liver is in fact due to amebas or to something else. Here a positive serology test will indicate that it *might* be due to amebas. A negative serology test will give one a 98% certainty that it is not due to the ameba. We must remember that the probability of a person having residual antibodies from previous infection depends also on his environment. Consequently one has to have, or should have, as absolutely essential information, some concept of the prevalence of antibodies in individual populations. Bear in mind that this information, the seroepidemiology of amebiasis, is probably the most accurate method we may have of estimating the importance of invasion by amebas in any area. It tells us nothing of the number of people who harbor amebas; it does tell us (or give us a concept) of the number of people whose tissues have been invaded by amebas, and I think this is much more valuable information than stool findings alone.

DR. KERRISON JUNIPER: My laboratory is now in the process of analyzing the results of studies of more than 5,000 serum samples from about 4,000 patients from hospitals in the Little Rock area. We have used the indirect hemagglutination (IHA) test as our main means of screening patients serologically for amebiasis, then performing complement-fixation (CF) tests and agar-gel (GEL) diffusion tests on positively reacting serum samples.*

The IHA test was considered clinically significant (positive) at titers of 1:128 or above. One patient with extraintestinal amebiasis had a positive IHA reaction at a titer of 1:262,144 but most of the titers of patients with amebiasis ranged from 1:128 to 1:8,192, with no significant difference between extraintestinal and invasive intestinal cases.

The CF test was considered clinically significant at titers of 1:16 or above. One patient with extraintestinal amebiasis had a CF test positive at a titer of 1:1,024, but most patients with amebiasis had titers of 1:16 to 1:256, with no significant difference between extraintestinal and invasive intestinal disease.

The agar-gel double-diffusion test was performed according to Crowle's microslide method on 10 microliter samples. Most patients reacting in this test showed at least two precipitin bands; one showed as many as eight when first seen.

Of 16 patients with extraintestinal amebiasis, 88% gave positive IHA, CF, and GEL tests. This somewhat low incidence of positive reactors (most reports list 95 to 98% positive) was caused by two patients with classical clinical findings of amebic abscess of the liver, but in whom all the serological tests were negative. The incidence of positive tests in intestinal amebiasis for the IHA, CF, and GEL tests respectively were as follows: 63 invasive cases—98, 85, and 86%; 28 noninvasive symptomatic cases—61, 56, and 54%; and 32 asymptomatic cases—58, 58, and 52%

---

*Parke-Davis and Company supplied axenically grown *Entamoeba histolytica* antigen for these studies.

Although the IHA test was the most sensitive one, more unexplained positive reactions were encountered with it and the test often remained positive for periods as long as one to two years after cure of the disease. The CF and agar-diffusion tests correlated better with the presence of clinically active amebiasis, and both tests tended to revert to a normal reaction within about six months after cure, with a few exceptions.

I have found these three serological tests to be exceedingly valuable in the clinical diagnosis of amebiasis. Because of its sensitivity, the IHA test can be used as a screening method for clinically significant amebic infection. A positive reactor should be considered a suspect, and appropriate intensive stool examinations should be obtained. It is important to realize that a negative serological test for amebiasis does not exclude active amebic disease; and that serological testing does not replace adequate examination of the stool. The CF and GEL tests are useful in assessing the clinical significance of a positive IHA reaction. These serological tests do not replace skilled clinical judgement, and patients should not be given antiamebic treatment simply because of a positive test.

DR. HEALY. Dr. Powell, would you like to say something of your broad clinical experience and its relation to serology?

DR. POWELL. I agree entirely with what has been said so far about the use of serology in amebiasis. The first point I should like to make, not just from the viewpoint of serology but for the diagnosis of amebiasis, is that the key to diagnosis is awareness. If you do not think of amebiasis as a clinician, you are not going to think about a serologic test. One must be aware of the possibility of amebiasis in a patient. The next point is that you must look at the patient from a clinical point of view. If the patient presents as a typical case of invasive amebiasis you are unlikely to need the serological test. Our present laboratory methods and other predecures for diagnosis are perfectly adequate. For example, I deplore waiting for serological results in order to be absolutely certain that you are dealing with a liver abscess which is clinically obvious and in need of urgent aspiration.

Nevertheless serology can be exceedingly helpful. I have no hesitation in saying that in the particular hospital in which I work we have so much amebiasis that the serological test for amebiasis is the most valuable and the most reliable serological test that we do for any disease in our area. There is no doubt that the serological methods now available for the diagnosis of amebiasis are both highly sensitive and highly specific for detection of past and present invasive disease.

I want to say a word from the clinician's viewpoint about the danger of titer levels. Clinicians are very apt to think that because one person has a much higher titer than somebody else that therefore he has more amebiasis. This is incorrect. The level of the titer is not necessarily an indication of the degree of tissue invasion, and it seems to us from our studies that people vary quite considerably. Some are high "responders," some are moderate "responders," some are low "responders," and just a few seem to be negative "responders" as far as their titers are concerned.

There is no doubt that antibodies may persist for a good many years after cure. Therefore the presence of a positive test on the serum of a patient does not necessarily indicate active infection, nor after therapy does it mean that treatment has failed. There is generally a slow fall in the titer level after successful treatment. The length of time for the fall depends, I think, on the initial height of the titer before treatment. If you start off with a very high titer, it takes longer, in general, for this to fall or become negative than if you start off with a low titer. Of course, what we need and do not yet have is a test which will indicate active infection as opposed to past or cured infection. Such a test would make life much simpler.

The last point I should like to make is that we do have a great need for a simple, quick test which can be done in all those regions of the world where sophisticated laboratory methods are not available. And I can assure you from my experience around the world that many of our present tests are not likely to be used very widely in areas of invasive amebiasis. The facilities just aren't there. We need, and we hope we are close to having, a simple test that clinicians can do and understand .

COMMENT FROM THE FLOOR.. In our hands the IHA test was not too useful in Malaysia because we found the positivity rate in some areas to be 30 to 40%. The other thing that wasn't emphasized was the use of the IHA test as an epidemiological tool. Through the years, people have done stool surveys and no one really has shown what these surveys mean in terms of invasive amebiasis. Yet here we seem to have a very quick, easy, odorless method for discovering whether an area is having invasive amebiasis or noninvasive amebiasis.

DR. ELSDON-DEW. We have done some fairly extensive seroepidemiological studies, not only on populations but on conditions. Let me first deal with the populations and then I shall give you some idea as to the kind of results we obtained locally in Durban and over a wider range in South Africa. In the paper I have already presented I refer to the apparent difference (I said apparent) in amebiasis in the white and black populations. This is reflected markedly in the serological results. A random hospital population of Bantu had approximately 16% positive. The Durban Bantu volunteer blood donors, a slightly higher social stratum than the general hospital patient, had 9% positive. The whites in Durban are less than 1% positive. Black donors in Johannesburg are between 1 and 2% positive. Blood donors in Cape Town, less than 1%. This is illustrative of the kind of information you get.

On a slightly different scale, I thought that it would be of value to study the serology of people of different origins under uniform living conditions. I had the opportunity to do this because the gold-mining companies in the Transvaal operate blood-transfusion services and they have many donors of varying origins. I therefore tested the specimens of blood from these people. I was able to classify them as to whether they were Xhosa, Zulu, Sotho, and all the other native tribes, in addition to categorizing them by their geographic origins. The people from Botswana (formerly Bechuanaland), showed an unexpectedly high prevalence of antibodies. Botswana is in a remote portion of the country. I made inquiries, and it appeared that amebiasis was indeed quite common there. Thus, as far as I was concerned, serology had uncovered an area where I did not know that amebiasis existed. This was illustrative of the use of seroepidemiology.

There are other aspects of seroepidemiology. In one of our early studies we were able to study patients who had ulcerative colitis. We did not have any patients of our own thus afflicted and so we had to test some from other areas. These proved completely, utterly negative. We had in the same group in the same series, many cases of Dr. Powell's, those of postamebic dysentery or postamebic colitis; they were 100% positive. So, seroepidemiology can be applied not only to people and places, but also to disease states.

QUESTION. I have two questions to put to you. Persons at the National Institutes of Health (NIH) who have been doing indirect hemagglutination tests for us in suspected liver abscess have said that a negative reaction may indicate very early development of an abscess, and one may have to repeat the test, perhaps a few weeks later. I should like to know what relations these possible false negatives have in the diagnosis of very early acute liver abscesses? What is the present state of development and the potential use of soluble antigen fluorescent antibody test (SAFA) in amebiasis? Could it be applied in a large scale screening by use of the fluorimeter?

DR. HEALY. Let me answer the second question myself first. There is a movement today in serology, as there has been in clinical chemistry, toward the development of automated procedures. The soluble antigen fluorescent antibody test is being evaluated by a number of laboratories. My laboratory is collaborating with Dr. Roy Taylor of Fort Sam Houston, Texas, in comparisons of the IHA and SAFA tests in amebiasis. I think unfamiliarity with the machine is one of the basic problems.

I think the concept of having automated procedures by which one can test a great many specimens and get faster, more reproducible results is at the very forefront of development in serology. Dr. Kenneth Walls of our Parisitology Section at the Center for Disease Control has successfully adapted one of the automated devices used in clinical chemistry (the Technicon Autoanalyzer) for complement fixation tests for some of the parasitic diseases. The extent to which the SAFA test will be used as a screening device as well as for diagnosis depends upon its widespread use and evaluation as to its sensitivity and specificity. I refer your first question about false negatives to Dr. Powell.

DR. POWELL. I think it all depends, really, how early your patients with the liver abscess are presented to you. By and large our African patients in Durban tend to present fairly late. In the case of gel diffusion-precipitin studies, if one studies early, initial sera on admission one finds about 98% positive. If one repeats the study 10 or 20 days later, then one may increase that positivity rate by about 1%.

DR. JUNIPER. Our number of cases is small, but we have had one patient with a liver abscess, with symptoms of only two weeks' duration who had a positive serologic test; another with symptoms of four weeks duration had a positive test. I do not recall any of our invasive-colon patients with a negative serologic test who had a positive one later. All of our patients have been positive or negative serologically

174

throughout the course of the illness. However, it is interesting that very frequently we do see a significant rise in titer two or three weeks after the initial specimen, particularly after the patient has been started on treatment. In a few instances when patients, for various reasons, have not been treated, we have seen a continued rise in titer over a period of a number of months.

DR. ELSDON-DEW. I am going to theorize a little. You have all seen pictures of amebas in hepatic tissue. I do not like to use the word "liver abscess" because the lesion is not truly a liver abscess; it is an area of necrosis. One of the main pathologic features is a lack of tissue response; this rather suggests that the human host does not recognize the ameba as foreign. Yet we obtain a positive serologic response. The only way I can explain this is by assuming that some of the amebas die and release antigenic material from within. I do not think the human body recognizes the outside of the ameba as foreign. Hence it may well appear that we have to wait for the ameba to die for an antigenic stimulus to result. I think amebas die rather quickly, some of them even in the intestine.

DR. HEALY. As a parasitologist I find it interesting that amebas can "colonize" in the liver and produce, in some cases, a very large tissue abnormality, the abscess, and yet not initiate antigenic stimulation sufficient to produce an antibody response. It may be that they do colonize, grow, and multiply, and do not die and release any antigen until the abscess is fairly well developed, but I do not know how fast the abscess grows.

DR. JUNIPER. The thing that worries me about our two serologically negative cases is whether we might be dealing with another cause of "aseptic" necrosis of the liver. I must admit that the patients responded very nicely to emetine treatment. This would seem to indicate that the disease was amebic, but it is conceivable that there might be another etiology. It astounds me that a negative serologic reaction can occur in the presence of an amebic abscess.

DR. POWELL. We have found E. histolytica in the aspirate in one or two serologically negative cases. But this is certainly very uncommon. As to the question of how long it takes to develop a liver abscess, I do not know the whole answer, but we have seen liver abscesses develop in babies five or six weeks old.

QUESTION. Dr. Powell: on the question of titer. If, as you point out, the higher titer is not necessarily a manifestation of greater tissue invasion, what should we take as a significant titer?

DR. POWELL. I think you have to work that out on the basis of the control in your local population. Dr. Healy showed some nice biphasic curves, and I think he found that for the local populations which these represented, a significant titer was 1:128.

DR. HEALY. I do not think one need be concerned about a diagnostic titer in too many instances. It has been my experience in the diagnostic laboratory that sera from cases of amebiasis, particularly liver abscesses, generally have fairly high IHA titers, much beyond the minimum level of 1:128, we established, as Dr. Powell indicated. Our minimum diagnostic titer is 1:128 based on seroepidemiologic evidence and clinical information in our original studies. We recently tested a serum, by IHA, from a young man in Florida who had a liver abscess. The titer of his serum, tested several times, fluctuated between 1:128 and 1:256. The physician aspirated a liter of pus from his liver. He responded very well to emetine. Such a low titer is unusual; the majority of sera from cases of severe clinical amebiasis are positive at titers of 1:1024-2048 and many 1:32,000 or greater.

QUESTION. Dr. Healy, would you suggest that two or more specimens be collected so that a rising titer might be detected?

DR. HEALY. No. As has been pointed out, it has been the experience of several workers that differences in titer are not apparent on all acute-convalescent status such as exists in virology or with some direct agglutination tests that are used in bacteriology. The same titer or a two-fold dilution difference may persist from a few weeks to several months or more and then drop slowly.

QUESTION. Will you discuss intradermal reaction in amebiasis?

DR. ELSDON-DEW. The intradermal reaction is testing something entirely different from what we have been discussing. It is not a test of circulating antibodies. We know that there is something happening but I do not think we really have adequate information yet. Frankly, when we have such easy tests as the serologic ones, I should say that we should use serologic rather than skin tests for now. Undoubtedly we shall learn more about skin-test reactions in due time and then be better able to answer that question properly. Dr. Powell raised a point a moment ago and I should like to comment on it here if I may.

We have studied the gel-diffusion test, in depth, to the extent of isolating the various antigenic fractions concerned. The gel-diffusion test suffers from one clinical disadvantage (it is not an epidemiologic disadvantage); that is, it takes a little time to complete gel diffusion. You have to wait for antibodies to diffuse toward the antigens and, in fact, one cannot report an unequivocal negative reaction in less than 48 hours. This is a clinical disadvantage. Another disadvantage is that a certain amount of technical expertise is necessary. The test is not something which can be done ad lib or "in the bush," so to speak.

In Durban we have been trying for a long time to find some simple method of serologic testing. We have developed a latex test which on comparison with the gel diffusion gave an agreement within 1%, which is as good, I think, as one may expect to get between two serologic tests. We are not absolutely sold on the present latex test as it is, and we are still awaiting reports on whether the test is really as good in other people's hands as it has proved in ours.

QUESTION. Dr. Elsdon-Dew, were your population studies done with the gel-diffusion test?

DR. ELSDON-DEW. Yes, all with gel diffusion.

DR. HEALY. I think that the serologic diagnosis of amebiasis is "coming of age," so to speak. The World Health Organization has lately become interested in evaluating the effectiveness of amebiasis serology on a global basis, and we have recently completed some studies in five countries. There are companies interested in marketing diagnostic kits, and commercial amebiasis antigens or test kits have shown great promise in preliminary work. These kits will be available, I am sure, because there has developed a keen interest in them and they are needed. At the present time I know of at least three companies who are testing commercial amebiasis antigens.

QUESTION. Has anyone done much work on children in terms of their titers? We found, and you confirmed this, Dr. Healy, that some of the children did not have a high rate of negativity in terms of titers as might be expected if one considers that they are primary responders rather than secondary responders.

DR. HEALY. I have not had any extensive experience with young children.

DR. POWELL. One of our pediatricians in Durban has been doing a study using gel diffusion and, in the case of liver abscesses, the percentage of positives in children in the same, or approximately the same, as in adults. In the case of amebic dysentery there is a far greater percentage of negatives in very young children. Children tend to approximate the percentage of positives in adults after four years of age. Certainly, in very young children, the percentage of positives is less.

DR. JUNIPER. From a slightly different aspect: whenever we have an individual with invasive disease, we try to obtain serum from all members of the family. Sometimes there are as many as 10 children in these families, and the incidence of positive reactors is very high. In some instances the sera from the entire family will react, whereas we may demonstrate *E. histolytica* in the stools of only one half the family members. However, I am impressed that children become seropositive to amebic invasion very readily.

QUESTION. I should like to ask about the standardization and origin of the antigens in view of the fact that in early isolates host red-cell antigen would be present. Is there an attempt to standardize antigens and perhaps indicate how long an ameba should be cultured before the antigen would be considered standardized?

DR. HEALY. Most of the ameba cultures used for growing organisms for antigens are quite old, and I do not believe there is any host antigen associated with them. For example, in our laboratory we are growing, in Diamond's axenic medium, the HK-9 strain of *E. histolytica* isolated in 1952. This strain was brought to this country by Dr. W. W. Frye in what I have been told was a very smelly flight because he had several culture tubes strapped to his body when he brought back the several K strains from Korea in 1952. I do not think many workers are growing amebas or using amebas for antigens directly isolated from a patient, either from stools or from liver abscess. Years ago investigators made antigen by alcoholic extract of amebas in liver abscess fluid or organisms from severe amebic dysentery, but today most people use antigens from amebas that are grown in culture without any host antigens.

QUESTION. Would you comment on the use of serology in amebic hepatitis.

DR. POWELL. I think it is an important one. One of the most valuable contributions that serology could make for us is in helping to delineate precisely what are the conditions of invasive amebiasis. I think that there are two most fertile fields for this. One is in delineating amebic hepatitis, if it exists as a condition, and the other is in helping us to sort out the vague condition of chronic, sympotomatic, internal, intestinal amebiasis which is another very variable diagnosis.

DR.VICTOR G. HEISER. It is customary at symposia such as these to call upon an old Methuselah who by personal experience can connect the distant past with the present. My experience with amebic dysentery began in 1902 in Egypt, then in India, and then, on a very large scale, in the Philippines.

We soon found that at the time the United States government had taken over the administration of the Philippines, large numbers of Americans were employed by the Philippine government. It is safe to say that nearly half these employees and their families developed dysentery, although not always amebic dysentery. Then we found that they had exactly the same experience in other countries. Other tropical countries showed the same incidence, the British in India, Malaya, and Borneo, the French in Indochina, the Dutch in Java, the Australians in New Guinea.

Another clinical characteristic developed. In most of these countries which were dominated by either Americans or Europeans, it was customary on the approach of the hot season, to move the government to higher altitudes. This was almost invariably accompanied by large outbreaks of epidemics of diarrhea; here again not necessarily all outbreaks were due to amebic dysentery. It is well to mention that in the early years, perhaps up until 1908, it was not recognized that there were pathogenic and nonpathogenic amebas. We recognize that today, of course. In the Philippines, standard treatment for amebiasis included a huge enema, frequently given daily, of quinine solution. This treatment took two to three weeks to cure a routine case. The other alternative was ipecac, so you can imagine how unpopular the treatment for amebic dysentery was. Then Sir Leonard Rogers came along with his reports of the success of emetine in treating amebic dysentery.

It may be of interest to mention that at the close of World War I it was anticipated that a large number of amebic cases would come back with the returning troops. In anticipation of this possibility, the Rockefeller Foundation organized a unit that was intended to deal with this problem should it occur. Fortunately the returning troops had very little dysentery and there was no need to use the facilities which the Rockefeller Foundation was prepared to make available.

# SYMPOSIUM ON CHOLERA

## Introduction*

### KEVIN M. CAHILL, M.D.

Director, Tropical Disease Center
St. Clare's Hospital and Health Center
New York, N. Y.

Professor of Tropical Medicine
Royal College of Surgeons
Dublin, Ireland

THIS seventh in the series of symposia in clinical tropical medicine again focuses on a disease that not only was but is of importance to physicians in temperate as well as in tropical climates. In fact cholera in many ways epitomizes the lurking potential of "tropical" infections in this jet age, changing within a short time from a smoldering endemic in far off Bengal to a fulminant epidemic encircling the world.

Cholera is again on the march. In the 1960's the El Tor biotype of the vibrio sprang from its Celebes origins, spread across Southeast Asia and, as the pandemic gained momentum, cholera suddenly exploded south of the Sahara for the first time in the recent history of Africa. Cholera became a major health problem in the last year in the Soviet Union, in

---

*Presented as part of a *Symposium on Cholera* sponsored by The Tropical Disease Center, St. Clare's Hospital, New York, N. Y., and The Merck Company Foundation, Rahway, N. J., held at the Center, June 5, 1971.

181

Israel, and in innumerable countries in the Middle East, with occasional introduced cases in Europe. The disease once again became a concern for the traveler and a priority item for public health officials as well as for the journalist, the politician, and the diplomat, all of whom had to deal with populations frightened by the specter of fatal diarrhea and the complications of restricting economic growth and tourist activities in already borderline "developing" areas. The recent devastations—flood and later military conflict—afflicting East Pakistan (Bangla Desh) were accentuated by cholera. Many refugees were infected, and it is estimated that more than 10,000 died from the disease.

The very word "cholera" evokes the image of quarantine ships, fumigating pots, and individual and community devastation. François Magendie said that cholera was "a disease that begins where other diseases end, with Death." From public panic for this single infection grew many of the health laws and departments that we know today. The history of cholera in the United States is reviewed in this collection by Dr. John Duffy, professor of the history of medicine at Tulane University. Dr. Duffy details the impact cholera had on New York as well as in the Mississippi Basin. The status of cholera around the world is considered by Dr. Eugene J. Gangarosa of the National Center for Disease Control, who is responsible for charting the current spread of the disease for our government. In addition to a concise review of the epidemiology of cholera he addresses himself to the specific questions of the threat of cholera to American travelers and of the potential hazard of introduced cholera in this country.

It is almost impossible to imagine the advances in our knowledge of the pathophysiology and clinical management of cholera in the past decade. My own introduction to this disease was in Calcutta in 1959 and, at that time, merely on the basis of a clinical diagnosis, hope was generally abandoned and patients were admitted to Mother Theresa's Hospice for the Dying where I worked; in fact, as soon as a diagnosis was confirmed in neighboring institutions patients would be transferred to the hospice since the mortality rate was so astronomically high and the potential threat of transmission so feared. In this symposium Dr. Thomas R. Hendrix reviews a number of the basic studies that now permit an understanding of the mechanisms underlying the incredible production of fluid in cholera feces—often between 70 and 75 liters in several days. These studies became the basis for improved clinical management.

The clinical studies Dr. Carpenter's group have done in Calcutta are classic, and he elucidates the approach in management that has resulted in a reduction of cholera mortality from 75% or more to less than 1% in properly treated patients. Dr. Richard Hornick's work on cholera in volunteer patients has permitted controlled observations in the prime animal model afflicted—man, and his careful study in the spirit of John Snow is entitled "The Broad Street Pump Revisited." The limitations of cholera vaccination, and the current dependence of control programs upon the availability of adequate amounts for fluid replacement are reviewed by Dr. Abram S. Benenson who was the director of the Southeast Asia Treaty Organization Cholera Research Laboratories in Dacca, East Pakistan, for five years. For anyone familiar with the devastation of the disease, the inadequacy of health services, and the lack of both personnel and equipment in the areas generally afflicted, this view by Dr. Benenson emphasizes the urgent need for continued research for better ways of controlling and preventing this disease.

Once again it has been our effort here to present the most up-to-date information on those aspects of an important worldwide disease of interest to the modern physician.

# THE EPIDEMIOLOGY OF CHOLERA: PAST AND PRESENT*

EUGENE J. GANGAROSA, M.D.

Deputy Chief, Bacterial Diseases Branch
Epidemiology Program
Center for Disease Control
Atlanta, Ga.

URING the past decade cholera has once again emerged from ob-
scurity. The current pandemic, the seventh, began in 1961 on
the island of Sulavesi (Celebes) in Indonesia. It is difficult to give a true
account of its spread and to define precisely the present situation in the
world because surveillance has been so incomplete and ineffective. During 1961-1965 the disease spread through most of Asia; in 1965-1969
it penetrated the Middle East; and during 1970 there was extensive
dissemination into Africa.

Despite the lack of information from certain countries, it is quite
clear that 1970 was the peak year of this pandemic so far. Outbreaks
occurred not only in previously reported endemic foci but also in such
countries as Korea and Brunei, which had been free of the disease since
1964. It spread significantly into the Soviet Union, Turkey, and Czecho-
slovakia. The epidemic was introduced into Guinea during the summer.
There it found ideal conditions for dissemination. It spread along the
West African coast and inland by way of the great rivers, especially
the Niger. Simultaneously, the disease extended from Asia into East
Africa. By the end of the year it had spread through large parts of
Africa (see accompanying table).

The cholera situation in the world in mid-1971 is depicted in Figure
1. It is apparent that recent foci pose a direct threat to the Western
Hemisphere. But how real is the risk? Is it just a matter of time before
the disease gains a foothold in the Americas? To appraise this risk we
must understand cholera, past and present.

*Presented as part of a *Symposium on Cholera* sponsored by The Tropical Disease
Center, St. Clare's Hospital, New York, N. Y., and The Merck Company Foundation,
Rahway, N. J., held at the Center, June 5, 1971.

## COUNTRIES PRESENTLY REPORTING CHOLERA: 1970-1971

| Geographic area | Presently infected* | Previously infected in 1970-1971 | Imported cases only |
|---|---|---|---|
| Asia | Burma India Indonesia Nepal Pakistan Philippines Vietnam | Brunei Malaysia Singapore South Korea | Japan |
| Middle East | Gaza Strip Syria Trucial Oman (Dubai) | Israel Jordan Kuwait Lebanon Saudi Arabia Turkey | |
| Africa | Cameroon Chad Dahomey Ghana Guinea Ivory Coast Kenya Liberia Mali Niger Nigeria Sierra Leone Somalia Togo Upper Volta | Afars and Issas (formerly French Somaliland) Ethiopia Libya Tunisia | |
| Europe | | France Czechoslovakia USSR | Wales (U.K.) |

*Reported by the World Health Organization for the week ending May 19, 1971.

## THE ETIOLOGIC AGENT

A thermolabile exotoxin elaborated by the bacterium *Vibrio cholerae* is responsible for the disease. The organism is a gram-negative, curved, rod-shaped bacterium which is actively motile because of a single polar flagellum. There are two biotypes, the "classical" and the El Tor. The latter is responsible for the present pandemic. It is a hardier strain than the classical strains responsible for past pandemics in that it persists longer in nature and in man. It is also more resistant to chemical agents.

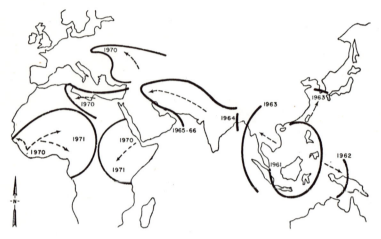

Fig. 1. Extension of El Tor cholera: 1961-1970. Source: *Principles and Practices of Cholera Control.* Revised according to *Weekly Epidem. Rec.: 45,* Nos. 1-52, 1970, and *46,* Nos. 1-23, 1971.

## RESPONSES TO INFECTION

Man is the only known reservoir in nature. There is a broad spectrum of responses to infection. The diagnosis of an overt case of cholera, cholera gravis, is relatively easy (Figure 2). Diarrhea can be so severe as to cause cardiovascular collapse and death in less than a day. Stool bicarbonate loss can lead to severe metabolic acidosis with Kussmaul breathing. Protracted vomiting further complicates the electrolyte and fluid imbalance. Depletion of potassium may result in impairment of renal and cardiac function. The patient often presents in shock with his clothes soiled by the voluminous feces. Although he may complain of severe abdominal and other muscle cramps, there is no tenesmus. The fecal discharge, which is not at all malodorous, is usually clear with flecks of mucus imparting a "rice-water" appearance. The skin has a doughy consistency; the hands are wrinkled as if long submerged in water, the so-called "washer-woman's hand" sign. Although phonation may be impaired, the patient is quite lucid.

But infection with the El Tor vibrio more often causes no symptoms or is so mild that it cannot be readily differentiated from other acute

186

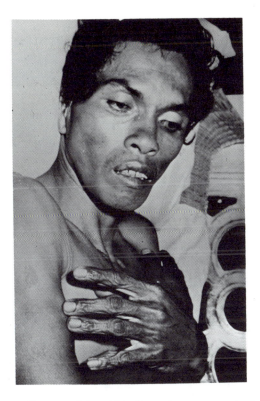

Fig. 2. Patient with severe cholera. Note the sunken eyes, prominent cheeks, and "washerwoman hand."

enteric illnesses. The case-to-infection ratio in classical cholera is about 1:7; in contrast there may be 25, 50, or even 100 mild or asymptomatic infections in the community for each severe El Tor case[1, 2] (Figure 3). These asymptomatic persons, some of whom may be incubating the disease, and those with mild illness may travel and take the disease with them, thus establishing new foci.

## TRANSMISSION

The disease normally spreads contiguously from one country to

187

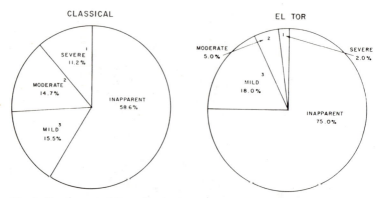

Fig. 3. Spectrum of cholera: distribution by per cent of individuals infected with classical versus El Tor cholera. 1) Hospitalized cases of cholera gravis; 2) cases detected in outpatient clinics; 3) cases detected in bacteriological surveys.

another. Traditionally, water routes have served as important routes of spread within a country and between distant countries. A new dimension of spread has been added in the present pandemic: importation of the disease by air travelers. This was probably the means of introduction of cholera into Guinea in the summer of 1970. During the past few years, cases have also been imported by air into Ghana, Japan, Australia, and England. In most instances, these importations were detected early because of better methods of surveillance of air passengers than of persons crossing land and sea frontiers. This is attributable in part to the better sanitary habits and higher living standards of air travelers compared with those of fishermen and land travelers. These three routes of spread—by land, sea, and air—make it practically impossible to prevent the introduction of cholera in even the most remote parts of the earth, but it is possible to prevent its spread and the great loss of life common in outbreaks in the past. This can be accomplished by setting up surveillance systems for diarrheal illness, by maintaining sanitary water supplies and sewerage, and applying modern treatment.

Cholera spreads only in a grossly unsanitary environment through contaminated water and food. The important role of water was recognized as early as 1854 by John Snow in his classic studies in London. With great precision, he recorded his observations and lucidly and convincingly described his conclusions:[3]

The pipes of each company go down all streets and enter nearly all quarters and alleys. A few houses are supplied by one company and a few by the other according to the decision of the owner or occupier at that time when the water companies were in active competition. In many cases a single house has a supply different from that on either side. Each company supplies both rich and poor, both large houses and small, there is no difference either in the conditions or occupation of the person receiving water from different companies. As there is no difference whatever, either in the houses or the people receiving the supply of the two water companies or in any of the physical conditions with which they are surrounded, it is obvious that no experiment could have been devised which would more thoroughly test the effect of water supply on the progress of cholera than this which circumstances placed ready made before the observer. The experiment too was on the grandest scale. No fewer than 300,000 people of both sexes, of every age and occupation, and of every rank and station from gentle folks down to the very poor were divided into two groups without their choice and in most cases without their knowledge; one group being supplied with water containing the sewage of London and amongst it whatever might have come from cholera patients, the other group having water quite free from such impurity.

Snow proceeded to demonstrate the dramatic differences in attack rates between cholera cases in homes supplied by the two water companies.

Southwalk and Vauxhall 71 per 10,000, Lambeth 5 per 10,000. Cholera was therefore 14 times as fatal at this period amongst persons having the impure water of Southwalk & Vauxhall Co. than amongst those having the purer water from Thames . . . it follows therefore that these houses (supplied by Lambeth) although intimately mixed with those of the Southwalk & Vauxhall Co. in which so great a proportion of mortality occurred did not suffer even so much as the rest of London which was not so situated.

This report is of great importance not only because of the demonstration of the role played by water in the transmission of cholera, but also because these observations could never have been made had there been significant spread by person-to-person contact. It is important to recognize that cholera, unlike shigellosis, is not easily spread by person-to-person contact. Physicians, nurses, ward attendants, and laboratory workers who have contact with cholera patients and their excreta almost never become clinically ill with cholera. Repeated examinations by culture of hospital attendants of cholera patients and neighborhood contacts in congested areas reveal that person-to-person spread is very rare indeed. This is because the inoculum required to cause clinical illness is extraordinarily large, a fact proved by volunteer studies.[4] Free in the environment outside its only natural host, man, *V. cholerae* is a fragile creature that succumbs promptly after desiccation and after a few days, even when kept moist. It is easily killed by chlorination and exposure to sunlight. Even when sources of water are heavily contaminated, vibrios spontaneously disappear in a few days after removal of cases or carriers. Thus, although water plays a major role in the transmission of cholera, the limited survival of the vibrio in water indicates that it cannot serve as a reservoir of infection. There is an important exception to this: cholera vibrios can survive long periods of time in sea water along beaches contaminated with human sewage. This is because of the affinity of these vibrios for salt water and the elimination of competing organisms by the high salt concentration.

Food has also served as an important vehicle of transmission. *Vibrio cholerae* will remain and even proliferate for several days in food which is alkaline and moist if competing organisms do not overgrow. Vibrios can remain viable for several days in moist clothing and bedding. These items were implicated by John Snow in the famous Broad Street pump outbreak.

Fomites, however, are not important in transmission. In recent outbreaks, extremely unwarranted measures were taken by some countries against the products of countries reporting cases. For example, in 1965 in the outbreak in Iran, Switzerland refused to accept Iran's mail and the Soviet Union banned shipments of chromate ore. There is no epidemiologic evidence to support these and numerous other measures often taken to restrict commerce from countries which report cases.

## Factors Contributing to the Pandemic

There appear to be several reasons why cholera has spread so dramatically since 1961. In recent years populations in developing countries have expanded so fast that their sanitation facilities and water supplies are taxed beyond capacity. Bad or nonexistent sanitation facilities permit fecal matter from infected persons to contaminate water supplies. Since *V. cholerae* is transmitted primarily by water, this contamination leads to the exposure of persons who drink the vibrio in water or use water for cooking or cleaning kitchen utensils. Further, the means and opportunities for travel have improved even for people in the developing countries, thus facilitating the spread of the disease by infected persons. Add to this a hardier strain known to cause more asymptomatic and mild diarrhea than the classical strain, and the stage is set for a pandemic.

### Risk to Traveling Americans

The immediate question that arises is: "How great is the risk to traveling Americans?" Well over half of the world's inhabitants now live in cholera-infected areas on three continents (see table). Literally millions of Americans and Western Europeans have traveled through or lived in these areas in the past decade. In that time there have been only four documented cases of cholera in American travelers, all nonfatal.[5-8] During the rapid geographic extension of the current pandemic in 1970, only one case of cholera was recorded in a traveler from a Western nation, England.[9] The risk is obviously small, much smaller than the risk of being injured in a car accident on the way to the airport. Thus it should not be necessary for anyone to cancel plans to travel anywhere in the world because of this risk.

### Protective Factors

Several factors account for this very low risk. Americans and other Westerners usually have standards of personal hygiene that minimize their exposure; they avoid questionable water and food supplies by frequenting tourist accommodations that tend to maintain high standards of sanitation. Second, Americans tend to travel within several weeks after being vaccinated against cholera, when vibriocidal titers are at a maximum. It is known that these titers correlate closely with cholera immunity[10] and that protection is greatest for the first two months after vaccination.[11] Finally, there are other nonspecific defense mechanisms, including the ability of gastric acid to kill enteric bacteria and the role of normal flora in eliminating competitors. Taken altogether, all of these factors constitute a formidable barrier against cholera.

Travelers should avoid eating uncooked vegetables, such as lettuce and celery, in cholera-infected areas, since these have been incriminated in outbreaks. Farmers are known to "freshen" their products on the way to market with water that may be contaminated. Fruits freshly peeled are quite safe. Bottled drinking water and soft drinks are generally safe. Swimmers should avoid beaches contaminated with human sewage, as the vibrios can survive for weeks in water with moderate salt concentration. If in doubt, they should swim only in constructed pools that contain chlorinated water.

### RISK FOR THE WESTERN HEMISPHERE

Another question that arises is: "What would be the risk of cholera transmission if it were introduced into the Western Hemisphere?" Air and sea traffic between cholera foci in West Africa or other cholera affected areas and American countries is increasing each year. The possibility of introduction of the disease has never been so great. The conditions necessary for transmission—highly susceptible populations crowded together under unsanitary conditions—exist in vast areas of Latin America. Ocean resorts contaminated with human waste, especially those in the warm, populous Caribbean area, are especially considered at risk. Some students of the disease predict that infection will spread in time to these parts of the Western Hemisphere.

The risk is quite different in the United States. Cholera is not transmitted in communities where water supplies are safeguarded and people ill with diarrhea use modern sanitary facilities. Since most areas have reasonably secure water facilities, the possibility of spread within the United States is considered quite remote. There are areas in the United States where sanitation standards are so low as to permit spread, but world travelers from such areas are so few that the possibility of introduction is minimal.

Surveillance efforts are being intensified. Health workers, hospital personnel, and laboratory supervisors are being contacted by various means to alert them to the problem. Physicians are being advised that they should consider cholera in the differential diagnosis for any patient who has diarrhea within five days after returning from an infected area. A rectal swab or stool culture should be taken and inoculated on solid agar or enrichment media. The specimen can be transported to the laboratory in Cary-Blair medium[12] or Sea-Salt medium[13] or, if these are not available, a piece of blotting paper dipped into the stool and sealed in a leak-proof plastic bag or screw-capped jar will do. The organism flourishes on readily available media such as MacConkey's agar but not on inhibitory media such as shigella and salmonella agar. Several highly selective media, such as thiosulphate citrate bile salts sucrose agar (TCBS) or tellurite taurocholate gelatin agar (TTGA), have been found very useful.[14] The diagnosis should be considered tentative until the organism has been definitely identified. Serologic tests are not valid for persons recently vaccinated against cholera. By international agreement all cases of cholera must be reported to the World Health Organization; therefore any proved or suspected case of cholera should be reported promptly to local and state health authorities and in turn to the Center for Disease Control.

## VACCINATION

Presently available cholera vaccines provide protection to only about 50% of vaccinated persons for no more than a few months, and they do not prevent transmission. In recognition of this fact and in consideration of the cost benefits, the surgeon general of the U.S. Public Health Service recently declared that this country will no longer require cholera vaccination for travelers coming to the United States from cholera-infected areas. He stated:

> There is clear evidence that cholera vaccine is of little use in preventing the spread of cholera across borders. We have, today, excellent treatment for cholera. The only effective method of preventing the spread of the disease is improvement of environmental sanitation. Therefore, in weighing costs and benefits, the United States has decided there is no reason for our government to require cholera vaccination as a condition of entry to the U.S. for travelers coming from an infected area. We believe strongly that this move benefits the better understanding of the disease at no cost to health.

Most other countries still require cholera vaccination for travelers. Accordingly, travelers should be vaccinated, ideally within two months of their anticipated departure. Although only one vaccination is required to fulfill international travel requirements, two vaccinations spaced one week to one month apart are strongly recommended. More than anything else, this ensures optimal freedom from most travel restrictions imposed by health authorities. Vaccination procedures and contraindications are detailed in an article by Gangarosa and Faich.[15]

## PROGNOSIS

Physicians should recognize that there is no longer any need for cholera to be thought of as a dread disease. Severe cases of cholera respond well to the intravenous fluid and electrolyte replacement therapy recommended by Carpenter and his associates.[16] Case-fatality ratios should not exceed 1%. Milder cases can be treated with either intravenous or oral fluid therapy[17] and tetracycline. Patients should be under enteric precautions in the hospital until the organism is no longer excreted in the stool, as proved by at least three consecutive daily stool cultures. Family contacts and others sharing the same eating and bathroom facilities should have stool cultures done but should not be quarantined. Tetracycline should be given for five days to contacts who are culture-positive and to those who are symptomatic, as recommended by McCormack and his co-workers.[18]

## SUMMARY

Cholera, a scourge of antiquity, has once again emerged as a major international health problem, but it should no longer be considered a dread disease because patients respond so dramatically to simple replacement of fluids and electrolytes. A new strain of *Vibrio cholerae*, the El Tor biotype, is responsible for the current pandemic. It is unique in that it causes so many asymptomatic and mild infections that are not easy to differentiate from a host of other acute enteric diseases. This property of the organism, the population explosion, and primitive sanitation—especially in the developing countries—the rapid means of transportation, and the lack of an effective vaccine account for its rapid spread by land, sea, and air on three continents in the past decade. The risk of cholera to the American traveler is very small, even less than the chances of injury in a car accident on the way to the airport. It is possible that cases will be imported into the United States, but the chances of spread within the country are very remote because of adequate safeguards of community water supplies. Physicians should think of cholera whenever a traveler-patient develops diarrhea within five days after returning from an infected area. Medical personnel should not be fearful of acquiring the disease because person-to-person contact transmission rarely, if ever, occurs.

## REFERENCES

1. Woodward, W. E., Mosley, W. H. and McCormack, W. M.: The spectrum of cholera in rural East Pakistan. I. Correlation of bacteriologic and serologic results. *J. Infect. Dis. 121*:S10-S16, 1970.

2. Bart, K. J., Huq, Z., Khan, M. and Mosley, W. H.: Seroepidemiologic studies during a simultaneous epidemic of infection with El Tor Ogawa and classical Inaba *Vibrio cholerae. J. Infect. Dis. 121*:S17-S24, 1970.

3. Snow, J.: *Snow on Cholera*, Richardson, B. W., editor. New York, Hafner, 1965.

4. Hornick, R. B. et al.: The Broad Street pump revisited. *Bull. N. Y. Acad. Med. 47*:1181-91, 1971.

5. Marr, W. L. and Gaines, S.: A possible case of mild cholera in an immunized American soldier. *Milit. Med. 129*:1061, 1964.

6. *WHO Weekly Epidem. Rep. 38*:570, 1963.

7. *WHO Weekly Epidem. Rep. 42*:364, 1967.

8. Abrutyn, E., Gangarosa, E. J., Forrest, J. et al.: Cholera in an American. *Ann. Intern. Med. 74*:228-31, 1971.

9. Editorial: Cholera again. *Brit. Med. J. 4*:2-3, 1970.

10. Mosley, W. H., Benenson, A. S. et al.: The relationship of vibriocidal antibody titer to susceptibility to cholera in family contacts of cholera patients. *Bull. WHO 38*:777-85, 1968.

11. Azurin, J. C., Cruz, A., Pesigan, T. P. et al.: A controlled field trial of the effectiveness of cholera and cholera El Tor vaccines in the Philippines. *Bull. WHO 37*:703-27, 1967.

12. Cary, S. G. and Blair, E. B.: New transport medium for shipment of clinical specimens. *J. Bact. 88*:96-98, 1964.

13. Venkatraman, K. V. and Ramakrishman, C. S.: A preserving medium for the transmission of specimens for the isolation of *Vibrio cholerae. Indian J. Med. Res. 29*:681-84, 1941.

14. Gangarosa, E. J. and DeWitt, W. E.: Laboratory methods in cholera: Isolation of *Vibrio cholerae* on TCBS medium in minimally equipped laboratories. *Trans. Roy. Soc. Trop. Med. Hyg. 62*:693-99, 1968.

15. Gangarosa, E. J. and Faich, G. A.: Cholera: The risk to American travelers. *Intern. Med. 74*:412-15, 1971.

16. Carpenter, C. C. J., Barua, D., Wallace, C. K. et al.: Clinical studies in Asiatic cholera. *Bull. Hopkins Hosp. 118*:165-68, 1966.

17. Cash, R. A., Nalin, D. R., Rochat, R. et al.: A clinical trial of oral therapy in a rural cholera treatment center. *Amer. J. Trop. Med. 19*:653-56, 1970.

18. McCormack, W. M., Chowdhury, A. M., Jahangir, N. et al.: Tetracycline prophylaxis in families of cholera patients. *Bull. WHO 38*:787-92, 1968.

# THE HISTORY OF ASIATIC CHOLERA IN THE UNITED STATES*

JOHN DUFFY, Ph.D.

Professor of the History of Medicine
Tulane University Medical School
New Orleans, La.

THE long history of the Western World has seen many diseases rise and fall. Leprosy, bubonic plague, sweating sickness, malaria, and smallpox at one time or another have all presented serious threats to the health of Europeans. The bubonic plague or Black Death swept into Europe in the mid-14th century, remained as an endemic disorder for 400 years, and then quietly disappeared. Smallpox became a major killer among diseases in the late 16th century, peaked in the 18th, and was already declining by 1796 when Jenner discovered vaccination. Diphtheria was of minor consequence prior to the 1730's and 1740's when it suddenly became widespread throughout Europe and eventually crossed the Atlantic to the American colonies. The last great pestilence to sweep through the Western World was Asiatic cholera, a highly fatal and terrifying disorder which came in three successive waves from 1832 to 1873. These cholera onslaughts coincided with and reinforced the 19th century movement for sanitation, the success of which guaranteed that the disease would never again plague an advanced industrial country.

Since the Atlantic Ocean has served as a transportation route rather than a barrier throughout most of American history, the endemic and epidemic disorders of Europe have invariably affected Americans. Malaria, typhoid, and a host of other infections landed with the first settlers. The one major difference in Colonial America arose from the relative isolation of the colonies from Europe and from each other. Many diseases which were endemic in Western Europe, such as smallpox and measles, did not gain a permanent foothold in America until the late 18th century. In consequence, for the American colonies they were major epidemic disorders, striking indiscriminately at persons of

*Presented as part of a *Symposium on Cholera* sponsored by The Tropical Disease Center, St. Clare's Hospital, New York, N.Y., and The Merck Company Foundation, Rahway, N.J., held at the Center, June 5, 1971.

all ages. As the population grew and trade with Europe increased, these infections also became firmly embedded in colonial towns and cities, and in so doing they became familiar complaints, no longer creating terror and alarm.

By the 19th century the eastern part of the United States was no longer a sparsely settled domain on the fringes of the Western World, but rather an integral part of it. Large urban populations and improvements in the land and water transportation systems had made certain that any new disease afflicting Europe would spread to and through North America. Moreover, the same urbanization and industrialization which set the stage for the relatively brief career of Asiatic cholera in Western Europe also had created a congenial milieu for it in North America. American cities were expanding too rapidly for the relatively weak municipal governments to cope with the growing sanitary and health problems. Effective sewerage and water systems were the exception for most of the century, and a good part of the town dwellers relied upon shallow wells fed by the constant overflow and seepage from the cesspools and privies. Perennial housing shortages resulted in jamming newcomers into dilapidated older dwellings left by the well-to-do as they sought newer and better housing on the outskirts. The crowded warrens occupied by the lower-income groups lacked all amenities and made personal hygiene virtually impossible. By 1832 the stage was set for the appearance of cholera in North America.

The background of Asiatic cholera, a disorder which had long been endemic in the Far East, is well known. Suffice it to say that a major outbreak in 1817 gradually spread westward. By 1830 it had reached Russia, and from there it swept through Europe to reach Great Britain by 1831. Early in the summer of 1832 the disease appeared in Quebec and Montreal and, shortly afterward, it spread to New York City. Asiatic cholera had all the properties for arousing fear and consternation. It was a new and unaccountable sickness; it coursed rapidly through the population; it could bring death in a matter of hours; and the pinched, blue faces and dark, drawn skin of its victims were a fearful sight to all who witnessed them.

The dread and apprehension caused by cholera was enhanced by the fact that it became the most widely heralded epidemic disorder ever to strike the United States. The advent of relatively cheap newspapers in the early 19th century provided an excellent medium for communication, and the American public was kept abreast of the seemingly inexorable spread of the disease westward. Long before cholera reached the United States, newspapers, popular magazines, and professional journals carried long, detailed accounts of its ravages in Russia and Europe. The intimate relation between dirt and disease was widely recognized, and editors, physicians, and private citizens all joined in urging local authorities to begin large-scale sanitation programs. By the time the epidemic wave reached England a rising air of tension and alarm was reflected in the news items and feature stories on cholera which were preoccupying the attention of American newspapers.

In the winter and spring of 1832 every American city began girding itself against the threatening pestilence. Mayor Walter Bowne of New York City proclaimed a strict quarantine against European and Asian ports, and the New York City Council formed a joint committee to suggest ways for improving the street-cleaning system. On June 15 news that cholera was present in Quebec and Montreal heightened the tension and stimulated the City Council to vote $25,000 for the Board of Health "to use in such manner as may be thought advisable, as the erecting of hospitals, and other means, to alleviate and prevent the cholera." The board promptly ordered city officials to enforce rigorously all health laws and to see that the city was made as clean as possible. At the same time the board sent two physicians to Montreal and Quebec to investigate the outbreaks there. In the meantime the local medical society organized a special 15-man committee to recommend preventive measures. The committee's recommendations, reflecting the prevailing medical beliefs, centered on a massive sanitation program, personal hygiene, and a moral and temperate life.[1]

By the time New Yorkers learned of the cholera outbreaks in Montreal and Quebec, the disorder had already entered upstate New York. The governor of the state promptly called a special session of the legislature. Within two days a health law was enacted and signed by the governor which provided for a strict quarantine along the Canadian frontier and required all towns and villages bordering on the lakes, rivers, and canals to appoint local health boards. Vermont and other states, too, began invoking quarantine measures and appointing temporary health boards.[2] As they had done for hundreds of years, the well-to-do citizens began a mass exodus from towns and cities, literally jamming the roads with their carriages and wagons.

By the middle of June cholera dominated the thoughts of New Yorkers. The subject became a favorite theme for sermons, and apothecaries began doing a land office business in cholera preventives. "The consternation in the city is universal," one New Yorker recorded in his diary on June 17, "Wall Street and the Exchange are crowded with eager groups waiting for the latest intelligence." [3] Despite the deplorable sanitary condition of the city, the Board of Health demonstrated a masterful inactivity and contented itself with reassuring the public that all was well. When several cases of cholera were reported by physicians late in June, the health officials refused to admit their presence. Since the announcement of the presence of a virulent epidemic disease often caused panic, health boards in this period were always reluctant to admit the fact until it was all too obvious. In this instance, with the wildest rumors spreading and the public already apprehensive, the Board of Health merely discredited itself. [4]

The reaction of New Yorkers to cholera had its counterpart in hundreds of other American cities and towns. In Pittsburgh the newspaper coverage of the cholera pandemic was similar to that of the New York journals. A series of articles in the winter of 1831-1832 discussed the cause, cure and prevention of cholera. Most writers emphasized that "intemperance, disorderly living, and want of cleanliness" were prime predisposing conditions, and they exhorted their readers to adhere "to a sober and temperate mode of living." In June 1832 the Pittsburgh *Gazette* editorialized that the spreading alarm was probably beneficial, since "there is great necessity for the most energetic measures for purifying our city. . . ." Pittsburgh had one major advantage, the *Gazette* added, in "the coal smoke which obscures our atmosphere while it neutralizes all the miasma which comes within its influence." Thus "the same furnace or factory which contributes to the luxurious enjoyments of the capitalist, saves the industrious laborer from the ravages of the disease." [5]

Far to the south the citizens of New Orleans were watching the course of the epidemic with a similar morbid fascination. The local newspapers were filled with stories of the progress of the disease and editorials and letters stressed the need for a drainage and sanitation program. The first direct impact of the arrival of cholera in the United States was felt by the local newspapers. The editor of the New Orleans *Courier* announced on July 17 that he was reducing publication to three times a week because the disruption caused by cholera in the North had cut his supply of paper and reduced the flow of news. On August 1 the *Courier* declared: "The Cholera continues to be the all absorbing topic of public attention. Reports of its progress are looked for by our citizens with intense anxiety. Go where you will, you hear nothing talked of but the *Cholera*—which seems to be thought worse than death itself."[6] Despite a series of scares, it was not until late in October that cholera arrived in New Orleans. Dr. Theodore Clapp, a prominent clergyman, claimed to have seen the first cases when he chanced upon two men in a dying condition who had been put ashore from a newly-docked steamboat. A crowd had gathered around them when a physician rode up, glanced at the men, and immediately declared they had Asiatic cholera. The crowd fled in panic. "That day," Dr. Clapp wrote, "as many persons left the city as could find the means of transmigration."[7]

Although New Orleans was the last major city to feel the effect of the disease in 1832, it suffered the heaviest casualties. Following the arrival of cholera late in October, the disease spread through the waterfront area with startling speed. On November 5 the New Orleans *Emporium* reported: "The people are in a state of suffering, despondency and excitement unparalleled in the history of our city. 'Death on the pale horse' for the last ten days has been rapidly engaged in the indiscriminate work of slaughter. Not less than *eighteen hundred* individuals have perished since the commencement of the disease." Corroborating the grim account of the *Emporium*, the *Courier* asserted four days later: "Since its commencement here it has made dreadful havoc, many believing that no less than 2,000 deaths occurred during the fourteen days commencing the 23rd October."[8]

Fortunately the outbreak lasted only a little over three weeks. In that period the estimates of the number of dead ranged from 4,350 to 5,000. This enormous mortality in so short a period of time created difficulties in burying the dead. A shortage of wagons and carriages was caused by the thousands who had fled to escape the successive epidemics of yellow fever and cholera, making it necessary for municipal officials to requisition all available vehicles to carry the dead to the graveyards. Even so, bodies accumulated at the cemeteries faster than they could be buried. Emergency measures, including mass burials, were put into effect, but occasionally as many as 100 bodies were waiting when the gravediggers arrived for work in the morning. The city's population of about 50,000 had been reduced to 35,000 by a yellow fever epidemic in the summer and early fall. Since it was further reduced by a second exodus following the appearance of cholera, this means that between 15 and 20% of the city's population was wiped out within less than a month. During this time virtually all economic activities were halted, and the task of caring for the sick and burying the dead preoccupied all who remained in New Orleans.[9]

In New York the outbreak lasted about six weeks; it reached a peak shortly after the middle of July and ended early in August. Here, too, the flight of so many middle- and upper-class residents brought economic stagnation, complicating the problems of the poor who invariably bore the brunt of the onslaught. The Board of Health spent $118,000 during this period; about 40% of these funds was devoted to a drainage and sanitary program and the rest for hospitals and medical care. Both the Board of Health and the Special Medical Council campaigned to raise the moral standards of the lower classes. Public notices advised personal cleanliness and temperance in eating and drinking, and urged workers to avoid laboring in the heat of the day. Just how men whose livelihood depended upon hard physical outdoor work could avoid the latter injunction was never stated; nor did anyone see the irony in advising the dozens of families sharing one hydrant and two or three privies to practice personal hygiene. Although the belated efforts of the Board of Health could have had only limited value, the death toll in New York was well below that in New Orleans. Nevertheless 3,000 of its citizens perished in the summer of 1832.[10]

The desultory fashion in which cholera took its toll is clearly illustrated in the case of Pittsburgh, Pa., and of Wheeling and Charleston, W. Va. The three cities exhibited the usual lack of sanitation and their citizens were justifiably apprehensive, yet none of these places suffered major outbreaks in 1832. A number of scattered cases led to 30 deaths in Pittsburgh in the late fall, but Wheeling and Charleston remained free of the disease. The latter city, however, had a narrow escape. A river boat with cholera aboard was wrecked on nearby Folly Island. When the infection spread to some of the residents, the authorities in Charleston immediately placed guards on the island to prevent anyone from leaving. Although over 50 cases and 20 deaths occurred on Folly Island, the rigid quarantine prevented the disease from spreading to

Charleston. The following spring, however, an explosive outburst in Wheeling brought death to 153 of the town's 3,500 inhabitants within the space of six weeks. In the small community of Triadelphia, eight miles east of Wheeling, cholera broke out in July of 1833 and within a few days there had been 17 cases and eight deaths in a total population of about 50. That same summer cases appeared in Pittsburgh and Charleston, yet in both instances did relatively little harm.[11]

As already noted, cholera started in upstate New York and from there literally spread throughout the eastern part of the continent. It followed the water and stagecoach routes to even the most remote communities, in some instances skipping lightly over a town or settlement and striking others with deadly effect. Of the major cities, only Boston and Charleston escaped the onslaught. In the South the disease proved devastating to Negro slaves. In coursing along the rivers and bayous it left an indelible impression wherever it landed. One Louisiana plantation alone lost 83 of its 104 slaves.[12]

As indicated, the disease continued to strike sporadically in 1833 and 1834 and then mysteriously disappeared for 15 years. The second great pandemic of Asiatic cholera reached the shores of America late in 1848 and ranged far and wide for seven years. The disorder had been general in Europe and Asia during the 1840's, and the mass migration of the Germans and Irish to America ensured that the infection would spread to the American continent. Like its predecessor, this epidemic wave was equally well heralded, and dire warnings were sounded by the newspapers and medical journals. The temporary health boards brought into existence by the previous outbreak had long since withered on the municipal vines, and the tentative efforts toward municipal sanitation had been swamped by the exploding city populations.

Sanitary conditions in 1848 were at least as bad as they had been when cholera first appeared. In those cities which provided street cleaning, the work was performed by private contractors who conscientiously and all too successfully sought to do as little as possible. Street cleaning contracts were considered a form of political patronage, a state of affairs scarcely conductive to clean streets. Hogs, with some assistance from dogs and cats, were the chief scavengers, but they added little to the cities, either aesthetically or in terms of health. In the preceding 15 years a few miles of sewerage had been added to the major cities, but much of the wastes continued to pour into the gutters, open streams, and canals.[13]

Under these circumstances, Asiatic cholera proved just as devastating as it had in the previous attack. In New York City the Quarantine Station first reported the disease in December. Prompt and effective isolation measures kept the disease from spreading into the city, although 61 cases resulted in 32 deaths before the situation was brought under control. In the succeeding months occasional cases of what was suspected as cholera were reported, but it was not until May that a definite diagnosis was made of several cholera cases in the Five Points district, one of New York's worst slum areas. Despite all efforts by city authorities, the outbreak slowly picked up momentum in June and reached a peak in July. By the time the epidemic was proclaimed at an end, October 1, the official death toll amounted to 5,071. The true figure may well have been much higher. One of the physicians who served wtih the Board of Health claimed that private practitioners reported only a fraction of their cases. He estimated that cholera struck between 18,000 and 20,000 individuals, of whom about 8,000 died.[14]

Sporadic cases of cholera kept recurring in New York City during the next five years, with minor outbreaks almost every summer. The disease broke out in epidemic fashion once again in the summer of 1854. The precise death toll is not clear, but 1,178 deaths were recorded from cholera as of August 11. Fortunately, the worst of the epidemic was over by this time. This attack marked the end of the second wave, and cholera virtually disappeared from New York for about 12 years.[15]

Almost at the same time that the pestilence landed in New York City, it appeared in New Orleans. Here, too, the source of infection was an immigrant vessel which arrived on December 18, 1848. Unlike New York, where the infection had sputtered and flared for several months before reaching epidemic proportions, in New Orleans an explosive outburst immediately spread throughout the city. One of the newspapers conceded that the disease had caused 800 deaths by the end of December, while Dr. Joseph Jones, a prominent local health leader, subsequently estimated a death toll of 1,641 during this two-week period. In the course of the following year another 3,176 deaths from cholera were recorded. The disorder continued to flare up every year through 1855, the annual cholera deaths ranging from 450 to 1,448. After 1855 only a few scattered cases were reported until 1866, when the disease again struck in epidemic fashion.[16]

During all of these years, the disorder swept up and down the rivers and bayous of Louisiana, causing justifiable alarm and inflicting heavy casualties. In the spring of 1850 a diarist in North Louisiana recorded: "Cholera prevailing on boats, many dying." Few towns and villages escaped the disease, but wherever the infection appeared, Negro slaves seemed to bear the brunt of the attack. Many planters sought to protect their slaves by moving them into the woods. In Alexandria, La., the local newspaper reported that the appearance of cholera had caused one plantation owner to send all 700 of his slaves into the pine woods. The action was taken too late, the editor added, since 70 slaves were already dead and another 80 sick with the disease. Bishop Leonidas Polk wrote from his plantation: "We were during the presence of the disease absolutely so occupied as hardly to have a moment for anything but attention to the sick and dying and so could do nothing in the way of advising our friends of our condition." Of the 300 odd residents on his plantation, only 50 had escaped the disease and 70 had died. Polk mentioned another plantation which had lost 97 slaves, "65 of whom died in the field three days after the attack was made."[17]

The Pittsburgh area and western Pennsylvania managed to escape most of the worst effects of the second wave of cholera. On New Year's Day, 1849, the Pittsburgh *Gazette* reported that cholera had struck New Orleans and was now moving up the Mississippi River. In this and succeeding issues, the editor suggested the establishment of a cholera hospital and urged the civic authorities to purify and cleanse the city. The disease reached Pittsburgh in March of 1850, striking in and around the city in desultory fashion. As summer advanced and the number of cases increased, a Pittsburgh newspaper stated: "A thousand vague rumors of the terrible ravages of the cholera are flying around town, and the minds of our citizens are filled with apprehension."[18] Fortunately, the worst fears were not realized, and by September the disorder subsided. From March to September the cholera death toll stood at 300. Sporadic cases were reported in the succeeding years, but the disease did not flare up epidemically until 1854. In that year it exploded late in July and early September and killed about 1,000 of the city's approximately 50,000 residents. This marked the last major assault on Pittsburgh.[19]

As had been the case during the previous outbreak, Asiatic cholera spread throughout the United States in 1849. The Western cities, with their large transient populations, took heavy casualties. St. Louis, Cin-

cinnati, Sandusky, San Antonio, and a host of smaller towns all experienced severe outbreaks of cholera, in some instances losing 10% or more of their populations. After 1849 the disease continued to flare up for six more years before finally burning itself out in 1854-1855.[20]

The third wave of cholera arrived in 1866, once again giving ample warning of its coming. By this date the relation between bowel discharges and the spread of the infection was generally recognized; moreover, the sanitary movement was in full swing. The net effect was to reduce drastically the impact of the disease. In New York the threat of cholera had helped propel a measure through the state legislature creating a Metropolitan Board of Health for New York City. This agency resorted to strenuous measures to clean the city and to identify and isolate cholera cases. Judging by the course of the epidemic in the rest of the country, New York City probably would have experienced only a mild outbreak, but the efforts of the health officials undoubtedly helped to minimize its effects even further.[21]

The infection once again coursed through America, but with a few exceptions the attacks were relatively mild and short-lived. New Orleans, which had endured a long military occupation and the resultant social and economic disruption, suffered heavily during this attack. The first cases were diagnosed in August 1866 and the disorder quickly spread throughout the city. On this occasion cholera exacted about 1,294 deaths. The disease returned the following year and claimed another 681 victims. In 1868, the last cholera year, only 129 deaths were reported.[22] It should be borne in mind that mortality figures for this period are always suspect; many deaths went unrecorded and even the best of physicians were often uncertain as to the cause of death. Cholera returned to the United States in a small way from 1873 to 1875. The presence or rumors of its presence created a considerable public furore, but the cases were few and scattered. Nonetheless, the threat of Asiatic cholera continued year after year to bring forth newspaper editorials and feature stories, to alarm the public, and to provide the sanitarians and health reformers with a rallying cry. Even as late as the 1890's the fear of cholera gave impetus to major public health reforms.

The medical profession was going through one of its most difficult times during the epidemics of Asiatic cholera. Revolutionary developments in science, technology, industry, and transportation were rapidly changing the Western World. In the field of medicine gross anatomy had been well delineated, pathological anatomy was established, microscopy was laying the basis for histology and cellular pathology, and developments in chemistry and physics were being applied to physiology; but all these advances seemed meaningless in terms of the one major preoccupation of medical practitioners: how to deal with the great epidemic diseases. The germ theory had been postulated in the 16th century, but it was only one of many medical theories. Even the question of whether diseases were distinct entities or merely manifestations of constitutional imbalances induced by meteorological and other environmental conditions was still not settled. Moreover, physicians were equally at odds over medical treatment. To make matters worse, the rising spirit of scientific inquiry had destroyed faith in traditional authorities, but was unable at this time to fill the vacuum it had created. Searching desperately for some sort of stability, practitioners grouped themselves around forceful individuals who set forth their theories with firm conviction. Inevitably these schools of medical thought clashed with each other. Not content with intellectual disputes, physicians publicly criticized their colleagues' medical practices and often resorted to bitter personal attacks.

The advent of Asiatic cholera found the profession completely divided over its cause and method of treatment. Their experiences with cholera in 1832 convinced most physicians that the disease was not directly communicable. They noted, for example, that attending physicians in the cholera hospitals rarely if ever came down with it. They also recognized that the disease flourished in the crowded and filthy slum areas. Early in the 1832 outbreak Dr. Alexander Stevens, president of the New York City Board of Health's Special Medical Council, reported that the disease was confined to "the imprudent, the intemperate and those who injure themselves by taking improper medicines. . . ."[23] Dr. Stevens' letter to the board illustrates one other characteristic of physicians in those days; few of them doubted that they could cure the disease provided the treatment was initiated at the first onset.

The divisions among New York physicians reflected the divergent medical practices of doctors generally. The Special Medical Council advised that the best therapeutics were calomel, opium, brandy, and cayenne pepper. The Kappa Lambda Society, a group of physicians organized primarily for social purposes, recommended as a preventive measure that patients be freely purged with calomel and aloes or scammony. Once the disease had set in, applications of heat, frictions and sinapisms were advised. Doses of medicine should be small, and "if thirst is urgent, cold or iced water, or ice in small quantities, is never injurious." In cases of collapse, hot enemas with laudanum and brandy were to be used. Another group of physicians issued a regular publication during the epidemic called the *Cholera Bulletin*. On July 23, 1832, the editor commented upon the widely differing modes of treatment, and sarcastically classified his colleagues into the Bleeders, the Calomel Band, the Opium Foragers, the Company of Stimulators, the Tobacco Brigade, the Saline Aparients, the Guard of Leechers and Blisterers, the Men of Friction, and the Icy Guard. Having contributed his own share to professional disunity, he blandly observed that too many doctors turn "the weapons that should be directed against the enemy towards their fellow 'filii Esculapii.' "[24]

In the intervening years between the first and second attacks of cholera, little progress was made, and the outbreak in 1848-1849 found the medical profession as divided as ever. Early in 1849 the city inspector for New York warned that the introduction of water from Croton had increased the dampness of the soil, a condition known to be conducive to cholera. The Board of Health's Special Medical Council reiterated the view expressed in 1832 that the cause of the disease lay in the atmosphere, but that it was usually brought on by "exciting causes" such as intemperance, inadequate diet, and so forth. The next month the Board of Health proclaimed that since "it has been incontestibly proved by sad experience that fish, fruits and vegetables, in a state of decomposition, are especially provocative of Cholera," the sale of these items from carts and wagons in the streets would be prohibited. The New York Academy of Medicine, after debating at great length, was unable to decide whether or not the disease was contagious.[25]

The New York Board of Health appointed a "Sanatory Committee" that included nine laymen and five prominent physicians to report on the 1849 epidemic. The committee explained that it did not intend to inquire into the causes, nature, or treatment of cholera, "feeling assured that if the members of [the medical] profession acknowledge themselves embarrassed by numerous problems connected with this mysterious disease" laymen can scarcely enter into it. The committee did conclude, however, that the disease was spread by the atmosphere. Dr.

William P. Buel, who had charge of two of the city's cholera hospitals, agreed with the committee, stating that he had found no evidence of contagion. His treatment consisted of administering opium by mouth and rectum to check the diarrhea. Since opium tended to reduce secretions, Dr. Buel compensated by prescribing camphor in chloroform. He added that tannin, "acetate of lead, nitrate of silver, sulphates of zinc, alumina and copper, were all used and with happy effects." The combination "of opium and acetate of lead, swallowed, or thrown in the rectum, forms a remedy of singular, and I think, unsurpassed efficiency." Illustrating what must have been a masterly balancing of his therapeutics, he wrote: "to restore suppressed secretions, calomel was, in the great majority of cases, administered, in combination with opium and astringents." His colleague, Dr. Alexander F. Vache, followed a similar regimen. It was Dr. Vache's judgment that "astringents and purgatives, copiously and promptly administered, are infinitely the best remedies." His preferred treatment was the use of tannin and calomel, combined with opium and camphor. "In the curable stages," he wrote firmly, "I do not doubt that the disease in most instances, will readily yield to these agents." Dr. Ovid P. Wells agreed with his colleagues, but he stressed the need to vary the treatment according to the needs of the patient. In serious cases he resorted to footbaths, "a strong infusion of capsicum," and mustard plasters to the stomach and abdomen. When fever supervened, he blistered the lower extremities, and cupped or leeched the abdomen, chest, and head.[26]

These same forms of therapy were used throughout the United States with occasional minor variations. A standard treatment on Louisiana plantations during the 1832 epidemic consisted of giving a large dose of calomel followed several hours later with a dose of castor oil. The old standby treatments, bleeding and blistering, were also resorted to as the disease progressed. One Louisiana physician wrote in 1855: "I have, for some years, prescribed cupping with as much confidence of success as a dentist would prescribe extraction for the tooth ache. I use the mercurial alterative merely to restore the secretions. The opium and astringent I use from habit. I commenced with them and have kept them up. I never use any medicine until the symptoms are relieved by counter-irritation." After describing what was obviously a rigorous form of therapy, the doctor stated with more truth than he realized that in cholera "as many die from excessive medication as die from disease." [27] A member of the Howard Association, a group of young business men in New Orleans who aided the sick in times of epidemics, wrote that his physician instructed him in a case of violent cramps "to give a salt and mustard emetic, to be followed by a dose of ten to twenty grains of calomel, afterward to keep the patient warmly covered in bed, and equalize the temperature of his body by mustard-baths or cataplasms on the extremities." [28]

In the 1830's a number of experiments were made with an intravenous infusion of a saline solution. In nearly all instances the patients were virtually moribund, and although they revived temporarily, death ensued shortly afterward. A Pittsburgh newspaper in reporting one of these experiments in the city's Cholera Hospital in 1834 suggested that the saline infusion might prolong life long enough for the victims to be able to make their wills and settle their earthly affairs.[29] Nothing came of the experiments, and the results seem to have discouraged any further attempts.

By 1866 the reliance on massive doses of calomel, castor oil, and other drastic remedies was giving way to a more moderate practice. Dr. Warren Stone, writing in the *New Orleans Medical and Surgical Journal* in 1866, reported his success in giving cholera patients as much ice water as they wished. He also struck a blow at the traditional practice of counterirritants: "One thing, I know, certain, and that is, that the nerves cannot be tortured into the performance of their functions any more than heretics or rebels. The torture of counterirritants, hot applications, and burning things in a stomach, that is already suffering the sense of heat, only serves to intensify the disease and confirm the collapse." [30] Heroic medical practices were to hang on for many more years, but Dr. Stone's viewpoint, which represented the attitude of the better physicians, shows that by 1866 the tide had already turned.

Regardless of the medical profession's views, the public never wavered in its belief that cholera was contagious. The first rumors of its presence was enough to start a mass exodus. With physicians and scientists in disagreement about the cause of cholera, state and municipal officials played safe by supporting both quarantine and sanitary measures. Whenever the disease threatened, city councils usually appointed a board of health or else assumed the powers and functions of a health board. The first action taken by these newly-created health boards was to proclaim a quarantine and to provide for the isolation of the sick.

The next step was to see that the sanitary regulations were resurrected and rigorously applied. Street-cleaning contractors, who looked upon their duties as nominal, suddenly found themselves denounced on all sides. Funds were appropriated to clean the streets, alleys, vacant lots, and other public areas, and special attention was paid to the discharges and refuse of the so-called "noisome" trades. Municipalities were forced to make some provision for the poor and the sick. Temporary cholera hospitals were established and, as they became crowded, not infrequently doctors and nurses were hired to care for the sick in their homes. The multitude of local health boards which came into existence during the first two waves of Asiatic cholera were temporary agencies designed to meet the emergency. Once the crisis was past, these boards were quickly disbanded.

The most notable change in the public reaction during the cholera years was the growing assumption that society could do something about epidemic diseases. During the first two waves of cholera the disease was equated with sin and poverty, two terms which were almost synonymous. Based on the assumption that God was punishing man for his wickedness, state and municipal authorities in the 1830's proclaimed days of fasting, prayer, and humiliation. A movement for one on the national level, however, was stoutly resisted by President Andrew Jackson on the grounds that such action would run counter to the American principle of separation of church and state. In 1849 Zachary Taylor had no such qualms and, with cholera striking a second time, he promptly declared a day of national prayer, fasting, and humiliation. By this time the sanitary movement was in full swing, and while government leaders still appealed for divine help, the major emphasis was upon self-help. The newly created temporary health boards were endowed with more money and more authority. Moreover, the presence of the disease for six or seven years kept these health agencies in operation for longer periods. The success of these boards in cleaning up many cities, combined with the fear of cholera, gave impetus to the movements for both health and social reform. The interrelation between poverty and disease was evident to all thoughtful men, and the outbreaks of cholera drove the lesson home.

By the third wave of cholera, 1866, municipal governments were beginning to assume responsibility for water, sewerage, and the collection of garbage, and the public was slowly coming to accept the idea that health, too, was of public concern. The threat of the 1866 epidemic was a decisive factor in the creation of the Metropolitan Board of Health for New York City. It strengthened the powers of the Louisiana State Board of Health, and in every state it lent credence to the arguments of the health reformers. The movement for improved health and sanitation was the product of many forces; what Asiatic cholera did was to dramatize the issue and help bring public health to the fore.

## NOTES AND REFERENCES

1. Duffy, J.: *A History of Public Health in New York City, 1625-1866.* New York, Russell Sage Foundation, 1968, pp. 282-84, 441-42.
2. Rosenberg, C. E.: *The Cholera Years.* Chicago, Univ. Chicago Press, 1962, pp. 23-24.
3. Rosenberg, C. E.: *The Cholera Years.* Chicago, Univ. Chicago Press, 1962, p. 22.
4. Duffy, J.: *A History of Public Health in New York City, 1625-1866.* New York, Russell Sage Foundation, 1968, p. 284.
5. Pittsburgh *Gazette,* October 18, November 18, 1831; June 26, 1832.
6. New Orleans *Courier,* July 17, August 1, September 15, 1832.
7. Clapp, T.: *Autobiographical Sketches and Recollections.* Boston, Phillips Sampson, 1857, p. 119.
8. New Orleans *Emporium and Daily Evening Journal,* November 5, 1832; the New Orleans *Courier,* November 9, 1832.
9. Duffy, J., editor: *The Rudolph Matas History of Medicine in Louisiana.* Baton Rouge, Louisiana State Univ. Press, 1962, vol. 2, pp. 138-41.
10. Duffy, J.: *A History of Public Health in New York City, 1625-1866.* New York, Russell Sage Foundation, 1968, pp. 285-87, 442.
11. Duffy, J.: The impact of Asiatic cholera on Pittsburgh, Wheeling and Charleston. *West. Pa. Hist. 47:*199-211, 1964.
12. Duffy, J., editor: *The Rudolph Matas History of Medicine in Louisiana.* Baton Rouge, Louisiana State Univ. Press, 1962, vol. 2, p. 142.
13. For illustration of this see Duffy, J.: Hogs, dogs and dirt: Public health in early Pittsburgh, *Pa. Mag. Hist. 87:* 294-305, 1963; and Duffy, J.: *A History of Public Health in New York City, 1625-1866.* New York, Russell Sage Foundation, 1968, Chap. 20.
14. *N. Y. J. Med. Collat. Sci. 3:*9-30, 1849; *4:*11-12, 10-17, 1850; New York City Inspector, *Annual Report,* 1849, 480-81, 501-03; *Report of the Proceedings of the Sanatory Committee of the Board of Health, In Relation to the Cholera as it Prevailed in New York in 1849,* New York, 1849, pp. 55-56.
15. Duffy, J.: *A History of Public Health in New York City, 1625-1866.* New York, Russell Sage Foundation, 1968, pp. 445-46.
16. Duffy, J., editor: *The Rudolph Matas History of Medicine in Louisiana.* Baton Rouge, Louisiana State Univ. Press, 1962, vol. 2, pp 143-45.
17. *Ibid.,* pp. 144-45.
18. Pittsburgh *Gazette,* August 5, 1850.
19. *Ibid.,* July 15-September 30, 1854; Wilson, E., *Standard History of Pittsburgh,* Chicago, 1898, p. 624; Gerberding, G. H., *Life and Letters of W. A. Passavant,* 6th ed., Greenville, Pa., 1906, pp. 264-65.
20. Rosenberg, C. E.: *The Cholera Years.* Chicago, Univ. Chicago Press, 1962, pp. 115-17.
21. Duffy, J.: *A History of Public Health in New York City, 1625-1866.* New York, Russell Sage Foundation, 1968, pp. 560-63.
22. Duffy, J., editor: *The Rudolph Matas*

*History of Medicine in Louisiana.* Baton Rouge, Louisiana State Univ. Press, 1962, vol. 2, pp. 443-44.

23. Communication from Special Medical Council to Board of Health, July 10, 1832. New York City Municipal Archives mss.

24. *Questions of the Board of Health, in Relation to Malignant Cholera. . . .* New York, 1832, pp. 3-6; *Report of the Committee of the K. A. Society . . . ,* New York, 1832; *Cholera Bull. 1,* July 23, 1832.

25. *City Inspectors' Reports,* vol. 1, 1836-1848, Document No. 43, Bd. of Aldermen, March 5, 1849, pp. 896-97; *New York J. Med. Coll. Sci. 3:*137-38, 1849; *Daily Tribune,* July 2, 1849.

26. *Report of the Proceedings of the Sanatory Committee of the Board of Health: In Relation to the Cholera as it Prevailed in New York in 1849,* New York, 1849, pp. 5-6, 8-9, 74-77, 85-88, 90-96.

27. Duffy, J., editor: *The Rudolph Matas History of Medicine in Louisiana.* Baton Rouge, Louisiana State Univ. Press, 1962, vol. 2, pp. 19-20.

28. Robinson, W. L.: *The Diary of a Samaritan.* New York, Harper, 1960, p. 84.

29. Pittsburgh *Saturday Evening Visitor,* August 23, 1834.

30. *New Orleans Med. Surg. J. 19:*18, 25-26, 1866-67.

# THE PATHOPHYSIOLOGY OF CHOLERA *

## THOMAS R. HENDRIX, M.D.

Professor of Medicine
Johns Hopkins University School of Medicine
Baltimore, Md.

### INTRODUCTION

A SIATIC cholera is an acute, severe diarrheal disease caused by the organism *Vibrio cholerae*. The clinical spectrum associated with infestation with this organism ranges, however, from asymptomatic carriers to fulminant disease leading to vascular collapse within two hours of the onset of symptoms.[1] The volume of stool passed in the course of the illness may be equivalent to or even exceed the patient's body weight. In a study of 12 consecutive cholera patients in Dacca, Pakistan, in 1964, Lindenbaum and his associates found that the average duration of diarrhea was 4.7 days (range 2.7 to 6.3) and that the stool volume passed during hospitalization averaged 30.8 l. (range 5.2 to 69.1), and this did not include stool passed prior to hospitalization.[2] In some outbreaks, untreated, the mortality rate may be as high as 60%.[3] Simply replacing fluid and electrolyte losses intravenously can reduce the mortality to less than 1%.[1]

Interest in the pathophysiology of Asiatic cholera is twofold. First, cholera is a major fatal infection in many of the world's most populous underdeveloped areas. Since the public health measures which resulted in eradication of cholera from Europe and America are unlikely to become operative in the endemic areas, better understanding of the disease may lead to the development of practical preventive and therapeutic measures; further, cholera has been a stimulus to reexamine intestinal secretion, a phenomenon that since the review of Florey et al.[4] has been largely ignored or was believed not to exist. (*The Handbook*

*Presented as part of a *Symposium on Cholera* sponsored by The Tropical Disease Center, St. Clare's Hospital, New York, N.Y., and The Merck Company Foundation, Rahway, N.J., held at the Center, June 5, 1971.
This study was supported in part by P.H.S. Research Grant AM 05095 from the National Institute of Arthritis and Metabolic Diseases and Grant AI08187 from the National Institute of Allergy and Infectious Diseases, Bethesda, Md.

*of Physiology*, which devotes five volumes to the alimentary tract, has not even a chapter on intestinal secretion.)

## THE INFECTION

Large numbers of *V. cholerae* are found in the stool in early cholera ($10^6$ or greater/ml. stool). Recent studies have shown that almost as many are to be found in the upper jejunum on the first day of illness.[5] In postmortem examination of fatal cases as well as in experimental infections of laboratory animals the organisms are found in large numbers "adsorbed" to the surface of the mucosa as well as in the luminal fluid.[6, 7] The organisms do not, however, invade the epithelium or enter the crypts of Lieberkühn.[8] The number of vibrio decreases in the small bowel as the diarrhea decreases and disappears on the fourth to eighth day of illness. A few patients continue to have vibrios in the small bowel even though the diarrhea has ceased. During cholera the upper bowel is colonized by colonic bacteria and these tend to persist, even for months after the acute illness.[5] It has been demonstrated in man and experimental animals that the clinical manifestations of Asiatic cholera are solely the consequence of the massive fecal losses of fluid and electrolytes.[1, 9, 10] This massive fluid and electrolyte loss can be duplicated by giving the bacterial-free filtrate of *V. cholerae* cultures to man[11] and experimental animals.[12-14] The active principle is an exotoxin which has been concentrated and purified so that nanogram amounts have biologic activity. It is a heat-labile protein with a molecular weight estimated to be between 10,000 and 90,000.[15, 16] Purification and characterization of the exotoxin have been hampered by the lack of a precise assay of its stimulation of intestinal secretion. The most precise tests of biologic activity, though indirect, are the capillary permeability test of Craig[17] and the release of glycerol by isolated fat cells.[18]

### SITE AND CHARACTER OF FLUID LOSS

The site of fluid loss in cholera is the small intestine in man and in experimental animals,[19-21] and fluid production is greater in the upper intestine, duodenum, and jejunum than in the ileum. There is no evidence that gastric, biliary, or pancreatic secretions contribute significantly to the cholera fluid. In experimental canine cholera 92.4% of the fluid produced comes from the jejunum and ileum while 5.6%

TABLE I. INTESTINAL FLUID COMPOSITION (mEq./l.)

| | | Jejunum | | | | Ileum | | |
| --- | --- | --- | --- | --- | --- | --- | --- | --- |
| | Na | K | Cl | HCO₃ | Na | K | Cl | HCO₃ |
| Man[24] | 148 | 5.6 | 138 | 15 | 146 | 5.7 | 121 | 42 |
| Dog[20] | 159 | 6.9 | 122 | 26 | 145 | 9.6 | 68 | 76 |
| Rabbit[21] | 153 | 4.3 | 45 | 92 | 148 | 4.4 | 48 | 91 |

comes from the alimentary tract proximal to the jejunum and 2% from the colon.[22] The colon continues to absorb fluid normally in cholera but because of its limited absorptive capacity it is unable to absorb but a fraction of the fluid delivered from the small intestine.[23]

The intestinal fluid in cholera is approximately isosmotic with plasma. Its electrolyte composition varies with the level sampled and from species to species but, more important, it is similar to the normal intestinal fluid for that species at that level (Table I).

The rice-water stool of cholera has a composition similar to ileal fluid (Na 139, K 24, Cl 106, HCO₃ 48).[2] The degree to which the electrolyte composition of stool is altered from ileal fluid is determined by the volume presented to the colon and the degree of hypovolemia and sodium depletion. The concentration of protein in cholera stools is very low, 85 mg./100 ml., well below levels found in congestive failure or inflammatory bowel disease.[25] In addition, after intravenous injection, neither Evans blue dye nor I¹³¹ labeled polyvinylpyrolidone appear in the stools of patients with cholera.

## MECHANISMS OF FLUID PRODUCTION

Having briefly reviewed the magnitude, composition, and site of production of the intestinal fluid that gives rise to the "rice water" stools of cholera let us review the mechanism by which it is produced. There have been four major suggestions: 1) exudation, 2) inhibition of absorption, 3) transudation, and 4) intestinal secretion.

*Exudation.* In view of the impressive evidence to the contrary it is surprising that this view of the pathogenesis of intestinal fluid production persisted so long. As recently as 1951 textbooks presented the views of Virchow and Koch that intestinal fluid losses were due to denudation of the intestinal epithelium; hence they could be likened to events seen after extensive burns.[26] In 1882 Cohnheim in his *Lectures on General Pathology* clearly pointed out that the choleraic stool had

215

such a low protein content it could not possibly be an exudate.[27] Although Goodpasture,[28] studying cholera in the Philippines, presented extensive histologic evidence in support of Cohnheim's view, the idea that morphologic alteration of the intestinal mucosa was a primary factor in the pathogenesis of cholera was not laid to rest until Gangarosa et al.[29] found normal intestinal mucosa by peroral biopsies during the course of cholera. Animal models of cholera have made it possible to follow intestinal morphology from first contact of the mucosa with *V. cholerae* or its exotoxin through to recovery.[8, 25] No light or electron microscopic alterations were found in the intestinal mucosa. In spite of the transfer of large amounts of fluid from mucosal capillaries to intestinal lumen only trivial changes if any could be found in the vascular or lymphatic vessels. These studies, as well as those in man, indicate that the intestinal fluid loss in cholera is mediated by a functional rather than an anatomical alteration of the intestine.

*Inhibition of absorption.* Using Visscher's calculations for the rate of clearance of sodium from plasma to gut lumen, Watten et al.[30] suggested that the explanation for the large fecal volumes produced in cholera was that the cholera organism or its products inhibit reabsorption of intestinal fluid. Support for this notion was provided by the observation that crude cholera toxin inhibited active sodium transport by frog skin.[31]

There are a number of reasons for rejecting this mechanism as the explanation for diarrhea in cholera. First, the application of Visscher's data to man probably overestimates the volume of fluid presented to the small intestine for reabsorption. It has been estimated that the small intestine absorbs 7 to 8 l. of fluid per day. Since there is no hypersecretion of saliva, bile, gastric, or pancreatic juice in cholera, complete cessation of intestinal absorption would result in a stool volume of no greater than 7 to 8 l. per 24 hours. On the other hand, the average stool volume observed in the first day of cholera was 8.3 l., and volumes as high as 16 l. have been observed.[32] Second, intestinal absorption of glucose is unaltered in experimental cholera.[33, 34] In fact, the normal glucose absorption in cholera has been put to practical use to increase fluid and sodium absorption from the intestine and to decrease the requirement for intravenous fluid replacement.[35, 36] Finally, measurements of unidirectional sodium fluxes both in man and experimental animals have shown normal lumen-to-mucosa movement of sodium with an increased mucosa-to-lumen movement.[24, 34, 37] Some observations have suggested that absorption of sodium may be decreased in cholera[37, 38] but, if present, it is not great and is not a major factor contributing to fluid and electrolyte losses in cholera.

*Transudation.* Intestinal fluid in cholera has a low protein content: hence it is not surprising that increased transudation into the intestine has been considered a mechanism for production of diarrhea in cholera. For such a mechanism to be operative, the hydrostatic pressure or driving force must be increased or the permeability of the mucosa increased (or, to put it in another way, the resistance to flow must be decreased) or there must be a combination of these two factors. Recently Love has presented data which have been interpreted as favoring increased mucosal permeability as the basic defect in cholera.[40] It was found that more fluid was drawn into the intestinal lumen by a similar osmotic gradient in the cholera-infected animals than in the normals. Calculations based on net fluid movement produced by unchanged solutes of varying molecular sizes lead to the conclusion that the effective radius of the epithelial pores of the intestine doubled (increased from a normal of 6 A. to 11-12 A.). Such calculations may have validity in the study of relatively homogeneous membranes such as frog skin or toad bladder but must be interpreted cautiously when applied to a complex epithelium like the intestine which has a heterogeneous population of cells and a secretory as well as an absorptive function. If the fluid and electrolyte response to cholera and hypertonic mannitol singly and in combination are measured it appears that the individual stimuli induce fluid of differing composition. When the two stimuli are given together the volume and composition of the fluid is what would be expected if the two stimuli were acting independently and their products were mixed.[41] When "free water clearance" is calculated for the mannitol-induced fluid in response to the combined stimuli no difference is found. If, however, cholera exotoxin had caused increased permeability of the mucosa more electrolytes could pass into the lumen and the free water clearance with the combined stimuli would have been less. Finally, if the movement of labeled noncharged solutes of varying size are injected intravenously and their appearance in intestinal fluid is measured, an estimate of mucosal permeability is obtained. Cholera does not alter the ratios, hence there is no evidence that cholera increases the permeability of the intestinal epithelium.[42]

There are other reasons for rejecting transudation as an important mechanism in the pathogenesis of cholera. In the absence of an osmotic gradient between the lumen and the lamina propria, the driving force for filtration through the epithelium is hydrostatic pressure. In cholera in man purging continues even when the patient is hypotensive and hypovolemic. In experimental canine cholera the rate of intestinal fluid production was not impaired when mesenteric blood pressure was decreased to 30% of control values by a clamp on the mesenteric artery.[43] The studies of Hakim and Lifson[44] are often quoted in support of the notion that hydrostatic filtration can explain fluid production in cholera. In these *in vitro* studies, net secretion was produced by increasing the pressure on the "serosal" surface. In this preparation net glucose movement was reversed when net fluid movement was reversed. In cholera, in contrast, glucose absorption continues at a normal rate as net fluid movement changes from absorption to secretion.[33]

Observations describing altered permeability and fine structure of the intestinal capillaries have also been used to support the hypothesis of transudation.[44-46] It has been reasoned that since permeability of the vessels of the skin is increased by injection of cholera toxin into the skin[17] cholera toxin may reach the intestinal vessels and produce similar changes. On the other hand, other observers have found no changes in the mucosal vasculature in experimental cholera.[8, 25] It seems reasonable to expect some functional changes in the mucosal capillaries in cholera since the large quantities of fluid appearing in the lumen are delivered to the epithelium by the mucosal capillaries. The likely interpretation of all this is that the vascular changes described are the response to and consequence of the massive intestinal secretion rather than the cause.[47]

Finally, neither increased epithelial permeability nor increased hydrostatic driving force can explain the differing anion concentrations found in the jejunum and ileum, which are similar to those found in the uninfected state and are characteristic of the fluid found in jejunum and ileum. Even if increased permeability were the explanation for the large volume of fluid entering the intestine, it would be necessary to postulate other mechanisms to maintain the constancy of the anion concentrations in the jejunum and ileum at concentrations differing considerably from plasma.

*Increased secretion.* Little has been written on intestinal secretion during the last three decades and, until recently, all fluid and electrolyte movements into the intestinal lumen had been assumed to be passive.[48] This view of normal intestinal physiology has, of course, greatly influenced the nature of hypotheses proposed to explain the pathogenesis of cholera. Physicians of earlier generations, however, held a different view. In 1855 Dr. John Snow suggested: "It would seem that the cholera poison, when produced in sufficient quantity, acts as an irritant on the surface of the stomach and intestine, or, what is still more probable, it withdraws fluid from the blood circulating in the capillaries, by a power analogous to that by which the epithelial cells of the various organs abstract the different secretions in the healthy body."[49] A similar view was held by Cohnheim, who concluded, after presenting extensive clinical, pathologic, and experimental data, that ". . . the process of cholera may be interpreted by supposing that first, under the influence of the virus, which has probably entered the intestine from without, there takes place, *an extra-ordinary profuse secretion from the glands of the small intestine.*"[50] Much evidence supports these suggestions that cholera fluid is the secretary product of the intestine.

First, in spite of the reversal of net fluid movement from "absorption" to "secretion" by cholera exotoxin, unidirectional flux of labeled sodium from intestinal lumen to mucosa as well as glucose absorption is unaltered from control values, whereas the flux of sodium from mucosa to lumen is greatly increased.[23, 34, 37] Such findings are difficult to reconcile with a passive process in the absence of any changes in physical driving forces such as hydrostatic and osmotic pressure.

Such consideration leads us to look for support for Cohnheim's hypothesis that cholera fluid originates in the crypts of Lieberkühn. If "absorption" and "secretion" are anatomically separated, cholera exotoxin might stimulate the "secretory area" while leaving the absorptive area unaffected. If cholera exotoxin stimulates secretion by the crypts of Lieberkühn without altering the absorptive function of the villi, agents which damage the crypts preferentially would be expected to modify the secretory response to cholera exotoxin. This notion was substantiated by studies of the effect of cycloheximide, an inhibitor of protein synthesis. On exposure to cycloheximide the epithelial cells of the crypts of Lieberkühn, having a higher protein synthetic rate, are effected earlier and at a smaller dose than are the columnar absorptive cells of the villi. The earliest morphologic evidence of the reversible inhibition of the synthesis of protein is disappearance of mitotic figures from the crypts of Lieberkühn. This reversible inhibition of maturation has been shown to be caused by inhibition of the synthesis of protein necessary for cells to go from prophase to metaphase. With increasing doses of cycloheximide the crypt epithelium shows irreversible damage, and eventually the epithelium of the villi show morphologic and functional abnormalities. At a level causing only disappearance of mitotic figures from the crypts, cycloheximide inhibits the outpouring of intestinal fluid that normally follows exposure of the intestinal mucosa to cholera toxin.[50] Calculations of bidirectional fluxes indicate that the cycloheximide effect is due entirely to inhibition of the exotoxin-induced increase in mucosa to lumen flux.[51]

Once the production of intestinal fluid has been instituted by cholera exotoxin, no inhibition by cycloheximide is evident until $2\frac{1}{2}$ to 3 hours after administration of the drug.[52] After cycloheximide the intestine does not regain its responsiveness to cholera exotoxin until protein synthesis recovers sufficiently to permit crypt cells to go into mitosis.[53] These findings suggest that cholera exotoxin induces the production of intestinal fluid through a process dependent upon protein synthesis. Once initiated, the secretion persists for several hours in the absence of further protein synthesis.

Another observation supporting the concept that the crypt and villous epithelia respond differently to cholera exotoxin is provided by measurement of the transmembrane potential by micropuncture of intestinal epithelial cells. The major changes induced by cholera toxin and theophylline (see below) were on the intervillous cells adjacent to the crypts and not on the villous cells.[54]

If the intestine is exposed to hypertonic sodium sulfate the villous epithelium is damaged, glucose absorption is impaired, but responsiveness of the mucosa to cholera exotoxin is unimpaired.[55] Finally, the newborn rat has no crypts and is unresponsive to cholera toxin. Production of intestinal fluid after exposure to cholera exotoxin appears only when the crypts of Lieberkühn are fully developed.[56]

Strong evidence that the production of intestinal fluid in cholera is the consequence of an active secretory process has been shown by studying intestinal mucosa in modified Ussing chambers. This permits measurement of unidirectional fluxes isolated from the effects of hydrostatic, chemical, and electrical gradients. In these experiments cholera exotoxin produced active secretion of chloride with a change in secretion of another anion, assumed to be bicarbonate, and with decreased sodium absorption.[39],[57] The differences between the *in vivo* and *in vitro* studies have yet to be resolved.

Most exciting is the observation that the *in vitro* effects on ion fluxes induced by cholera toxin were similar to those produced by cyclic AMP and by theophylline which causes endogenous cyclic AMP to accumulate by inhibiting its degradation by phosphodiesterase.[58] In addition, prostaglandins (PGA$_2$ and PGE$_1$) which also elevate tissue levels of cyclic AMP also lead to intestinal secretion. Intestinal mucosal levels of cyclic AMP have been found to be elevated by cholera exotoxin.[60] Recent studies have shown that cholera exotoxin activates adenyl cyclase in mucosal epithelial cells,[61] and it has been found that the level of intestinal adenyl cyclase in intestinal biopsies taken during acute cholera were twice the levels found in the convalescent period.[62]

Some of the pieces of this cholera jigsaw puzzle are beginning to fit together. The binding of cholera toxin to the intestinal epithelium sets off a sequence of events that results in the secretion of a characteristic isotonic fluid. One step in the sequence appears to be the activation of adenyl cyclase which, in turn, produces cyclic AMP; this provides the energy for the active ion transport which carries the fluid into the lumen. It also appears that there is an anatomic separation of absorptive and secretory function. The suggestion is that the choleraic fluid is produced by the crypts of Lieberkühn. There are, however, many missing pieces to find and fit into the puzzle. Where is the toxin bound? How are the secretory orders transmitted to the cell? Is activation of adenyl cyclase the primary event or is it the consequence of other events? Present information suggests that the onset of secretion precedes cyclase activation.[61],[63] What is the secretary process that is turned on? Is it the same in the jejunum as in the ileum? If chloride is indeed the ion that is secreted into the lumen in response to cholera toxin how are we to explain the excess bicarbonate in the luminal fluid?[21],[39],[64] The list can be easily extended manifold.

Finally, is the secretion of cholera a pathologic process or is it instead the extreme stimulation of a normal function? Is it a manifestation of what Florey et al.[4] suggested in their review of intestinal secretions:

> It may be necessary for a constant secretion of fluid to take place from the crypts of Lieberkühn to keep food particles in suspension while they are attacked by pancreatic enzymes, and

as the products of digestion are absorbed water and salts go with them. One may envisage a circulation of fluid during active digestion, the secretion passing out from the crypts of Lieberkühn into the lumen and back into the villi.[65]

## R E F E R E N C E S

1. Gordon, R. S., Jr., Feeley, J. C., Greenough, W. B., III, Sprinz, H. and Oseasohn, R.: Cholera. *Ann. Intern. Med.* *64*:1328-51, 1966.
2. Lindenbaum, J., Greenough, W. B., III, Beneson, A. S., Oseasohn, R. O., Risvi, S. and Saad, A.: Non-vibrio cholera. *Lancet 1*:1081, 1965.
3. Phillips, R. A.: Cholera in the perspective of 1966. *Ann. Intern. Med.* *65*:922-30, 1966.
4. Florey, H. W., Wright, R. D. and Jennings, M. A.: The secretions of the intestine. *Physiol. Rev.* *21*:36-69, 1941.
5. Gorbach, S. L., Banwell, J. G., Jacobs, B., Chatterjee, B. D., Mitra, R., Brigham, K. L. and Neogy, K. N.: Intestinal flora in Asiatic cholera. II. The small bowel. *J. Infect. Dis.* *121*:38-45, 1970.
6. Pollitzer, R.: Cholera. WHO Monograph series 43. Geneva, WHO, 1959.
7. Freter, R.: Studies of the mechanisms of action of intestinal antibody in experimental cholera. *Exp. Biol. Med.* (Suppl. 1) *27*:299-316, 1969.
8. Elliott, H. L., Carpenter, C. C. J., Sack, R. B. and Yardley, J. H.: Small bowel morphology in experimental canine cholera. A light and electron microscopy study. *Lab. Invest.* *22*:112-20, 1970.
9. Carpenter, C. C. J., Mondal, A., Sack, R. B., Mitra, P. P., Dans, P. E., Wells, S. A. Hinman, E. J. and Chaudhuri, R. N.: Clinical studies in Asiatic cholera. II. Development of 2:1 saline: lactate regimen. Comparison of this regimen with traditional methods of treatment, April and May 1963. *Bull. Hopkins Hosp.* *118*:174-96, 1966.
10. Sack, R. B. and Carpenter, C. C. J.: Experimental canine cholera. I. Development of the model. *J. Infect. Dis.* *119*:138-49, 1969.
11. Benyajati, C.: Experimental cholera in humans. *Lancet.* *1*:140-42, 1966.
12. De, S. N., Ghose, M. L. and Sen, A.: Activities of bacteria-free preparation from *Vibrio cholerae. J. Path. Bact.* *79*: 373-80, 1960.
13. Sack, R. B. and Carpenter, C. C. J.: Experimental canine cholera. II. Production by cell-free culture filtrates of *Vibrio cholerae. J. Infect. Dis.* *119*:150-57, 1969.
14. Finkelstein, R. A., Norris, H. T. and Dutta, N. K.: Pathogenesis of experimental cholera in infant rabbits. I. Observations on the intraintestinal infection and experimental cholera produced with cell-free products. *J. Infect. Dis.* *114*:203-16, 1964.
15. Coleman, W. H., Kann, J., Iwert, M. E., Kasai, G. J. and Burrows, W.: Cholera toxins: Purification and preliminary characterization of ileal loops reactive type 2 toxin. *J. Bact.* *96*:1137-43, 1968.
16. Finkelstein, R. A. and LoSpalluto, J.: Production of highly purified choleragen and choleragenoid. *J. Infect. Dis.* *121*: 563, 1970.
17. Craig, J. P.: Preparation of the vascular permeability factor of *Vibrio cholerae. J. Bact.* *92*:793-95, 1966.
18. Vaughn, M., Pierce, N. F. and Greenough, W. B., III.: Stimulation of glycerol production in fat cells by cholera toxin. *Nature* (London) *226*:658, 1970.
19. Banwell, J. G., Pierce, N. F., Mitra, R. C., Brigham, K. L., Caranasos, G. J., Keimowitz, R. I., Fedson, D. S., Thomas, J., Gorbach, S. L., Sack, R. B. and Mondal, A.: Intestinal fluid and electrolyte transport in human cholera. *J. Clin. Invest.* *49*:183-95, 1970.
20. Carpenter, C. C. J., Sack, R. B., Feeley, J. C. and Steenberg, R. W.: Site and characteristics of electrolyte loss and the effect of intraluminal glucose in experimental canine cholera. *J. Clin. In-*

*vest. 47:*1210-20, 1968.

21. Leitch, G. J. and Barrows, W.: Experimental cholera in the rabbit ligated intestine: Ion and water accumulation in the duodenum, ileum and colon. *J. Infect. Dis. 118:*349-59, 1968.

22. Sack, R. B., Carpenter, C. C. J., Steenberg, R. W. and Pierce, N. F.: Experimental cholera: A canine model. *Lancet 2:*206-07, 1966.

23. Greenough, W. B., III, Carpenter, C. C. J., Bayless, T. M. and Hendrix, T. R.: The Role of Cholera Exotoxin in the Study of Intestinal Water and Electrolyte Transport. In: *Progress in Gastroenterology,* Glass, G. B., editor. New York, Grune & Stratton, 1970, vol. 2, pp. 236-51.

24. Banwell, J. G., Pierce, N. F., Mitra, R., Caranasos, G. J., Keimowitz, R. I., Mondal, A. and Manji, P. M.: Preliminary results of a study of small intestinal water and solute movement in acute and convalescent human cholera. *Ind. Med. Res. 56:*633-39, 1968.

25. Morris, H. T. and Majno, G.: On the role of the ileal epithelium in the pathogenesis of experimental cholera. *Amer. J. Path. 53:*263-79, 1968.

26. Gradwohl, R. B. H., Benitez Soto, L., and Felsenfeld, O.: *Clinical Tropical Medicine.* St. Louis, Mosby, 1951, pp. 483-84.

27. Cohnheim, J. F.: *Lectures on General Pathology. A Handbook for Practitioners and Students.* Section III. *The Pathology of the Digestive System.* McKee, A. B., translator. London, New Sydenham Soc. 1890, pp. 949-60.

28. Goodpasture, E. W.: Histopathology of the intestine in cholera. *Philippine J. Sci. 22:*413-24, 1923.

29. Gangarosa, E. J., Biesel, W. R. Benyajati, C., Sprinz, H. and Pryaratn, P.: The nature of the gastrointestinal lesion in Asiatic cholera and its relation to pathogenesis: A biopsy study. *Amer. J. Trop. Med. 9:*125-35, 1960.

30. Watten, R. H., Morgan, F. M., Songkhla, Y. N., Vanikitai, B. and Phillips, R. A.: Water and electrolyte studies in cholera. *J. Clin. Invest. 38:*1879-89, 1959.

31. Fuhrman, G. J. and Fuhrman, F. A.: Inhibition of active sodium transport by cholera toxin. *Nature* (London) *188:*71-72, 1960.

32. Carpenter, C. C. J., Barua, D., Wallace, D. K., Mitra, P. P., Sack, R. B., Khanra, S. R., Wells, S. A., Dans, P. E. and Chaudhuri, R. N.: Clinical studies in Asiatic cholera. IV. Antibiotic therapy in cholera. *Bull. Hopkins Hosp. 118:*216-29, 1966.

33. Serebro, H. A., Bayless, T. M., Hendrix, T. R., Iber, F. L. and McGonagle, T.: Absorption of d-glucose by rabbit jejunum during cholera toxin-induced diarrhea. *Nature* (London) *217:*1272-73, 1968.

34. Iber, F. L., McGonagle, T., Serebro, H. A., Luebbers, E., Bayless, T. M. and Hendrix, T. R.: Unidirectional sodium flux in small intestine in experimental canine cholera. *Amer. J. Med. Sci. 258:*340-50, 1969.

35. Hirschhorn, N., Kinzie, J. L., Sachar, D. B., Northrup, R. S., Taylor, J. O., Ahmad, Z. and Phillips, R. A.: Decrease in net stool output in cholera during intestinal perfusion with glucose-containing solutions. *New Eng. J. Med. 279:*176-81, 1968.

36. Pierce, N. F., Banwell, J. G., Mitra, R. C., Caranasos, G. J., Keimowitz, R. I., Mondal, A. and Manji, P. M.: Effects of intragastric glucose-electrolyte solution on water and electrolyte enterosorption in Asiatic cholera. *Gastroenterology 55:*333-43, 1968.

37. Love, A. H. G.: Water and sodium absorption by the intestine in cholera. *Gut 10:*63-67, 1969.

38. Phillips, R. A.: Asiatic cholera (with emphasis on pathophysiologic effects of the disease). *Ann. Rev. Med. 19:*69-80, 1968.

39. Field, M.: Intestinal secretion: Effect of cyclic AMP and its role in cholera. *New Eng. J. Med. 284:*1137-44, 1971.

40. Love, A. H. G.: Permeability characteristics of the cholera infected small intestine. *Gut 10:*105-07, 1969.

41. Halsted, C. H., Bright, L. S., Luebbers, E. H., Bayless, T. M., and Hendrix, T. R.: A comparison of jejunal re-

sponse to cholera toxin and to hypertonic mannitol. *Hopkins Med. J.* In press.

42. Scherer, R. W., Harper, D., Banwell, J. G. and Hendrix, T. R.: Absence of concurrent permeability changes in intestinal mucosa with secretion. *Gastroenterology 60*:801, 1971.

43. Carpenter, C. C. J., Greenough, W. B., III and Sack, R. B.: The relationship of superior mesenteric blood flow to gut electrolyte loss in experimental cholera. *J. Infect. Dis. 119*:182-93, 1969.

44. Sheeby, T. W., Sprinz, H., Angerson, W. S. and Formal, S. B.: Laboratory *Vibrio cholerae* infection in the United States. *J.A.M.A. 197*:321-26, 1966.

45. Goldstein, H. B., Merril, T. G. and Sprinz, H.: Experimental cholera. Morphologic evidence of cytotoxicity. *Arch. Path. 82*:54-59, 1966.

46. Dalldorf, F. G., Keusch, G. T. and Livingston, H. L.: Transcellular permeability of capillaries in experimental cholera. *Amer. J. Path. 57*:153-170, 1969.

47. Hendrix, T. R. and Banwell, J. G. Pathogenesis of cholera. *Gastroenterology 57*:751-55, 1969.

48. Hendrix, T. R. and Bayless, T. M.: Intestinal secretion. *Ann. Rev. Physiol. 32*:139-64, 1970.

49. Snow, J.: *On the Mode of Communication of Cholera,* 2d. ed. London, Churchill, 1855.

50. Serebro, H. A., Iber, F. L., Yardley, J. H. and Hendrix, T. R. Inhibition of cholera toxin action in the rabbit by cycloheximide. *Gastroenterology. 56*:605-11, 1969.

51. Grayer, D. I., Serebro, H. A., Iber, F. L. and Hendrix, T. R.: Effect of cycloheximide on unidirectional sodium fluxes in the jejunum after cholera exotoxin exposure. *Gastroenterology 58*:815-19, 1970.

52. Harper, D. T., Jr., Yardley, J. H. and Hendrix, T. R.: Reversal of cholera exotoxin induced jejunal secretion by cycloheximide. *Johns Hopkins Med. J. 126*:258-66, 1970.

53. Banwell, J. G., Harper, D. T., Jr., and Hendrix, T. R.: Unpublished observations.

54. Hirschhorn, N. and Frazier, H. S.: Electrical potential profile of rabbit ileum: Effects of theophylline and chol-era exotoxin. *J. Clin. Invest. 50*:45a, 1971.

55. Banwell, J. G., Roggin, G. M., Yardley, J. H. and Hendrix, T. R.: Observations indicating cholera-induced secretion originates from the crypts of Lieberkühn. *J. Clin. Invest. 50*:5a, 1971.

56. Bayless, T. M., Luebbers, E. and Elliott, H. L.: Immature jejunal crypts: Absence of response to stimulus for fluid secretion. *Gastroenterology 60*:762, 1971.

57. Field, M., Fromm, D., Wallace, C. K. and Greenough, W. B. III: Stimulation of active chloride secretion in small intestine by cholera exotoxin. *J. Clin. Invest. 48*:24a, 1969.

58. Field, M., Plotkin, G. R. and Silen, W.: Effects of vasopressive theophylline, and cyclic adenosine monophosphate on short circuit current across isolated rabbit ileal mucosa. *Nature* (London) *217*:469, 1968.

59. Greenough, W. B. III, Pierce, N. F., Al-Awqati, Q. and Carpenter, C. C. J.: Stimulation of gut electrolyte secretion by prostaglandins, theophylline and cholera exotoxin. *J. Clin. Invest. 48*:32a, 1969.

60. Schafer, D. E., Lust, W. D., Sucar, B. and Goldberg, N. D.: Elevation of adenosine 3', 5' cyclic monophosphate in intestinal mucosa after treatment with cholera toxin. *Proc. Nat. Acad. Sci. 67*:851, 1970.

61. Sharp, G. W. G. and Hynie, S.: Stimulation of intestinal adenyl cyclase by cholera toxin. *Nature* (London) *229*:266-69, 1971.

62. Chen, L. C., Rohde, J. E. and Sharp, G. W. G.: Intestinal adenyl-cyclase activity in human cholera. *Lancet 1*:939-941, 1971.

63. McGonagle, T. J., Serebro, H. A., Iber, F. L., Bayless, T. M. and Hendrix, T. R.: Time of onset of cholera toxin in dog and rabbit. *Gastroenterology 57*:5-8, 1969.

64. Moore, W. L., Jr., Bieberdorf, F. A., Morawski, S. G., Finkelstein, R. A. and Fordtran, J. S.: Ion transport during cholera-induced ileal secretion in the dog. *J. Clin. Invest. 50*:312-18, 1971.

65. Florey, H. W., Wright, R. D. and Jennings, M. A.: The secretions of the intestine. *Physiol. Rev. 21*:36-69, 1941.

# THE BROAD STREET PUMP REVISITED: RESPONSE OF VOLUNTEERS TO INGESTED CHOLERA VIBRIOS*

R. B. Hornick, M.D., S. I. Music, M.D., R. Wenzel, M.D.,
R. Cash, M.D., J. P. Libonati, Ph.D., M. J. Snyder, Ph.D.,
and T. E. Woodward, M.D.

Division of Infectious Diseases
University of Maryland School of Medicine
Baltimore, Md.

THE Broad Street water pump in London was a source of cholera in 1854 as Snow[1] so carefully demonstrated. Snow's work implicated the important role water played in the spread of cholera. He postulated that contaminated water contained some form of viable contagion. Koch[2] was able to verify this hypothesis 30 years later by identifying vibrios from stools of patients with cholera in Egypt and India. The lack of an animal model has inhibited the acquisition of knowledge dealing with infectivity of vibrios. Carpenter et al.[3] have demonstrated many important facts in the pathogenesis of cholera with their canine model. However, the dog is markedly resistant to cholera infection and requires large numbers of organisms to induce disease.[3] Cholera is an enteric disease unique to man. In an effort, therefore, to evaluate vaccines a human model has been developed. This ability to study the induction of cholera in volunteers has established the postulates of Snow and Koch regarding the infectivity and virulence of *Vibrio cholerae* for man. This presentation will deal with results of studies conducted in volunteers infected with varying doses of classic cholera strains.

## Materials and Methods

Volunteers in these studies were inmates at the Maryland House of Correction. A well-equipped medical ward has been maintained for 10 years at the prison by the Division of Infectious Diseases of the Uni-

*Presented as part of a *Symposium on Cholera* sponsored by The Tropical Disease Center, St. Clare's Hospital, New York, N. Y., and The Merck Company Foundation, Rahway, N. J., held at the Center, June 5, 1971.

This investigation was supported by Contract No. 69-2002 of the National Institutes of Health, Bethesda, Md.

versity of Maryland School of Medicine. Several other enteric and viral respiratory diseases have been studied in this unit. The willingness and eagerness of volunteers to participate in all of these investigations is greatly appreciated and admired. The general plan of the cholera studies has been approved by the Cholera Advisory Committee of the National Institutes of Health. The Committee for Clinical Investigations at the University of Maryland School of Medicine has approved the protocols utilized in the studies. Each volunteer was informed of the nature of the disease and study plan and given several opportunities to withdraw prior to challenge. Appropriate laboratory studies including electrocardiogram, chest x ray, hematology, and blood chemistries were complementary to the histories and physical examinations in the selection of healthy volunteers.

Two strains of *Vibrio cholerae* were employed: Inaba 569B and Ogawa 395, two classic biotypes. Each had been used in the canine model and generously supplied by Charles C. J. Carpenter. The challenge organism was cultured on Brain Heart Infusion Agar (BHIA) overnight at 37°C. Identity was tested with group and type specific antisera, and 20 to 30 colonies were picked and suspended in BHIA. Preincubated BHIA plates were incubated with the BHI suspension. After 5 to 6 hours of incubation each plate was harvested with 5 ml, sterile buffered to $pH$ 7.2 + 0.1 with one part $M/15$ Sorensen's phosphate buffer to three parts saline. The harvested organisms were centrifuged in the cold at 2,500 RPM for 10 minutes. The pellet was resuspended and washed twice in four times the original volume. The suspension was standardized spectrophotometrically, and appropriate dilutions were made to approximate the organism count required for each challenge. Buffer-saline suspensions of the vibrio were made and the challenge organisms were always contained in 1.0 ml. Each inoculum was not only diluted and plated out for enumeration of the inoculum size but, after challenge of volunteers (usually within two hours), a repeat count of the inoculum was carried out to determine if any dying off had occurred between the laboratory manipulations and the time of challenge at the prison. Only those protocols in which adequate reproducibility of pre- and postcounts occurred were accepted for inclusion in the results presented here.

The challenge was conducted by placing the organisms in approximately 30 ml. of water which was then ingested by the volunteer. In

TABLE I. RESPONSE OF VOLUNTEERS TO VARYING DOSES OF
*VIBRIO CHOLERAE:* INABA 569B STRAIN (NO BUFFERING)

| Dose | Carrier | Diarrhea | | Cholera diarrhea | |
|---|---|---|---|---|---|
| $10^4$ | 0/2 | 0/2 | | 0/2 | |
| $10^6$ | 0/4 | 0/4 | | 0/4 | |
| $10^7$ | 0/4 | 0/4 | | 0/4 | |
| $10^8$ | 0/4 | 2/4 | 50% | 0/4 | |
| $10^9$ | 0/2 | 1/2 | 50% | 0/2 | |
| $10^{10}$ | 0/1 | 0/1 | | 0/1 | |
| $10^{11}$ (Bouillon) | 0/2 | 1/2 | 50% | 1/2 | 50% |
| Totals | 0/19 | 4/19 | 21% | 1/19 | 5% |

Evidence of cholera in 5/19 men: 26%

some studies 2 gm. of sodium bicarbonate in 60 ml. of water was administered just prior to the vibrios. All volunteers were fasted for two hours prior to and after the feeding.

Attempts were made to culture all stools from each volunteer. They were plated directly on Smith's Gelatin Agar (GA) and TCBS media (thiosulfate citrate bile salt sucrose). Subculture was to NGP broth and then into TCBS and MacConkey's agar. All suspect colonies were picked and inoculated into Triple Sugar Iron Agar and tested against antisera by agglutination.

Close clinical appraisal of each volunteer was maintained. Detailed fluid intake and output charts were kept on each individual. When it became apparent that stooling was at a rapid and increasing rate with a lag in oral intake, therapy with intravenous Plasmalyte* was begun. Adequate intravenous fluid was administered to maintain positive balance of fluid. Tetracycline therapy was administered to most of the volunteers who developed cholera diarrhea. In addition all other volunteers received 1 gm. of tetracycline per day for five days prior to discharge from the study.

## RESULTS

A wide spectrum of illness occurred after ingestion of varying doses of vibrios. For clarity of presentation of data, the various gradations

*Travenol Co. Contents: sodium 140 mEq./l.; potassium 10 mEq./l.; chloride 103 mEq./l.; acetate 47 mEq./l.; lactate 8 mEq./l.; calcium 5mEq./l.; magnesium 3 mEq./l.

TABLE II. RESPONSE OF VOLUNTEERS TO VARYING DOSES OF
*VIBRIO CHOLERAE:* INABA 569B STRAIN (WITH NaHCO₃)

| Dose | Carrier | Diarrhea | Cholera diarrhea |
|------|---------|----------|------------------|
| $10^1$ | 0/2 | 0/2 | 0/2 |
| $10^3$ | 3/4 | 0/4 | 0/4 |
| $10^4$ | 2/13 | 9/13 69% | 0/13 |
| $10^5$ | 1/8 | 5/8 63% | 1/8 13% |
| $10^6$ | 1/23 | 14/23 61% | 6/23 26% |
| $10^8$ | 0/2 | 1/2 50% | 1/2 50% |
| Totals | 7/52 13% | 29/52 56% | 8/52 15% |

Evidence of cholera in 44/52 men: 85%

of infection were classified as follows: *no evidence of infection:* i.e., negative stool cultures and lack of serological response; *carrier state:* the group of volunteers who manifested evidence of infection because of one or more isolations of *Vibrio cholerae* from stool cultures; *diarrhea:* those volunteers with at least one liquid stool containing the etiological organism but never requiring intravenous administration of fluid; and, finally, *cholera diarrhea:* volunteers with severe watery diarrhea requiring IV fluid to maintain fluid balance.

Tables I through IV indicate the frequency of these forms of cholera. The results demonstrate the common occurrence of diarrhea in the challenged volunteers. Some of these men had only a few liquid stools—a condition which would not cause one to seek medical attention. Total stool output measurements in this group ranged from 150 cc. to 42.9 l. Most of the men had 4 to 6 l. total volume of vibrio positive liquid stool. Figure 1 is an example of this mild form of cholera. Usually the diarrhea lasted seven days if untreated with tetracycline.

None of the volunteers with cholera diarrhea became severely dehydrated since intravenous fluid therapy was begun promptly when oral intake failed to balance output. A typical example of induced cholera diarrhea is shown in Figure 2. Note the early minimal diarrhea which began about 24 hours after challenge. Accelerated liquid stooling became apparent after 2½ days and reached a maximum rate on the third day. Tetracycline therapy and intravenous fluid was begun at this point and the rate of almost 1,200 cc. of stool per hour fell quickly, so that

TABLE III. EFFECT OF STOMACH BUFFERING ON INCIDENCE OF CHOLERA INFECTION

| Strain | Bicarbonate | Dose | Diarrhea | | Cholera diarrhea | |
|--------|-------------|------|----------|---|------------------|---|
| Inaba | 0 | $10^8 >$ | 4/8 | 50% | 1/8 | 13% |
| Inaba | + | $10^4 >$ | 29/46 | 63% | 8/16 | 17% |
| Inaba | 0* | $10^3$ | 2/9 | 22% | 0/9 | |

*Intraduodenal challenge

by 48 hours the rate was less than 100 cc. and by three days the diarrhea had ceased. The total stool volume in this man was 42.5 l. over a seven-day period.

Incubation periods on the mild diarrhea and cholera diarrhea was 47 to 36 hours respectively. In about 70% of the cases these initial stools yielded *Vibrio cholerae;* however, formed stools culturally positive for the vibrios were noted in 19% of the volunteers and, conversely, 12% of volunteers had liquid stools which failed to demonstrate vibrios upon culture.

Cholera in the volunteers had incubation periods which varied inversely with dose—the larger the dose, the shorter the incubation period.

Table I summarizes the experience with strain 569B in volunteers when administered without any buffering. These are washed organisms in pure culture (in the hope of reducing the amount of preformed toxin ingested). Nineteen men received from $10^4$ to $10^{10}$ organisms. No evidence of altered stool characteristics or isolation of vibrios occurred until a dose of $10^8$ organisms was swallowed. The two men who were given $10^{11}$ organisms had simultaneous beef bouillon in order to give a medium in which the vibrios could survive in the gastrointestinal tract. In these 19 men only 26% demonstrated some evidence of cholera, which indicated that healthy American males were not exquisitely sensitive to cholera. Many reasons for this apparent lack of susceptibility exist. A few will be mentioned here. First the strain of Inaba 569B was a laboratory-adapted strain that had been isolated in 1964 and that had many dog and rabbit passages prior to introduction to man. To obviate a possible loss of human virulence the organisms isolated from the volunteer who developed cholera diarrhea was utilized as a source of vibrios

Table IV. RESPONSE OF VOLUNTEERS TO VARYING DOSES OF
*VIBRIO CHOLERAE:* OGAWA 395 STRAIN WITH ($N_A$HCO$_3$)

| Dose | Carrier | Diarrhea | Cholera diarrhea |
|---|---|---|---|
| $10^3$ | 0/2 | 1/2 | 0/2 |
| $10^6$ | 0/22 | 11/22 | 9/22 |
| | 0/24 | 12/24 50% | 9/24 38% |

Evidence of cholera in 21/24 men: 88%

for subsequent studies. No obvious enhancement of virulence with this human isolate was noted.

Other factors involved in this host-parasite interaction include specific and nonspecific defense mechanisms. Cholera is not an endemic disease in this country and it would seem unlikely our volunteers would have the opportunity to develop immunity to cholera. They would be lacking in protective antibodies. Serum antibody data will be presented later but no evidence existed to suggest these men had significant humoral antibodies.

Nonspecific immune mechanisms are poorly understood. Acidity of the stomach has long been considered the first line of defense against many enteric infections, especially cholera. Table II demonstrates the enhancement of the virulence of vibrios by the addition of a buffering agent to the inoculum. Note that $10^4$ organisms was sufficient to induce diarrhea and that active cholera occurred after 100,000 vibrios. Increasing the dose of organisms produced a greater number of volunteers with cholera diarrhea while the proportion of mild cases of diarrhea remained the same. Over-all evidence of cholera was detected in 85% of the volunteers. Thus only 15% of those men ingesting bicarbonate and organisms were able to eliminate the ingested vibrios. However, it is of interest that even after 1,000,000 organisms about 9% of volunteers had no evidence of infection. Temporary carrier states occurred in 13%. Asymptomatic individuals such as these could be a source of further cases of cholera.

Table III compares the attack rates of cholera in volunteers infected with Inaba 569B with and without bicarbonate or directly into the duodenum. The addition of bicarbonate lowered the number of organ-

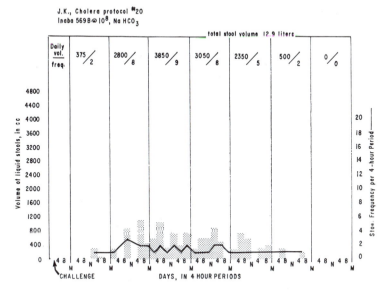

Fig. 1. Mild diarrhea.

isms required to cause disease from $10^8$ to $10^4$ organisms. These data suggested that the stomach was an effective barrier to further infestation by vibrios. Placing the organisms beyond the stomach did not result in any clear-cut conclusion but in at least two of these nine men the $p$H of the duodenal contents was acid and in one was alkaline. Perhaps the acid effect was not completely bypassed by introducing the tube from the stomach into the duodenum. The persisting acidity in the duodenum would be capable of inactivating the organisms.

Table IV outlines the virulence of Ogawa 395 in man. There was a suggestion that this strain caused more severe disease in the volunteers than Inaba; however, additional evidence is needed to confirm this trend.

The mechanism (or mechanisms) involved in the synergistic effect of bicarbonate was investigated in volunteers. Estimation of the $p$H of gastric contents was chosen as the simplest parameter to measure in man. The day prior to challenge a nasogastric tube was placed in the

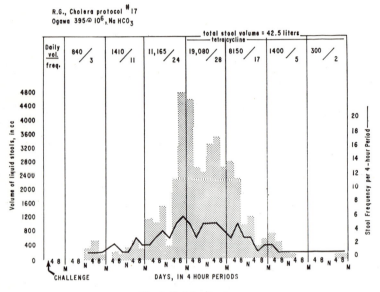

Fig. 2. Cholera diarrhea.

fasting volunteer. Stomach contents were aspirated every 15 minutes until 5 samples were collected. Two grams NaHCO₃ in 50 to 60 ml. of distilled water were drunk and four more samples were collected at 15-minute intervals. The $pH$ of each sample was determined with a Beckman $pH$ meter. In 36 men the contents of the stomach were acid prior to bicarbonate with the usual $pH$ less than 2.0. Analysis at 15-minute intervals of the $pH$ change revealed two distinct groups. One: the stomach contents were buffered to $pH$ 5.0 or greater; two: acid secretion in the second group rapidly overcame the buffering effect and the $pH$ returned to basal acid levels. The pharmacological effect of bicarbonate on gastric acid is a dynamic process. Immediately after the ingestion of bicarbonate probably all the men had a significant buffer effect. The duration of this presumed buffering action was less than 15 minutes in nine men. At 30 minutes 50% of this group had lost the measured buffering effect. By 45 minutes approximately 80% had returned to basal acid level, and no significant buffer effect was found at 60 minutes.

TABLE V. DOSE-SPECIFIC ATTACK RATES IN SECRETOR AND
NONSECRETOR GROUPS

| | 15 minutes after NaHCO₃ | | 30 minutes after NaHCO₃ | |
| | Secretor | Nonsecretor | Secretor | Nonsecretor |
| --- | --- | --- | --- | --- |
| $10^4$ | 1/4 = 25% | 4/5 = 80% | 1/5 = 20% | 4/4 = 100% |
| $10^6$ | 2/4 = 50% | 12/13 = 92% | 5/7 = 71% | 9/10 = 90% |
| $10^8$ | 1/1 = 100% | 1/1 = 100% | 2/2 = 100% | — |
| | 4/9 = 44% | 17/19 = 90% | 8/14 = 64% | 13/14 = 93% |

Cholera vibrios are exquisitely sensitive to low $pH$. The 15- and 30-minute postbicarbonate $pH$ determinations of the volunteers were correlated with the attack rates of disease. The group of men characterized as overcoming the bicarbonate effect was termed "secretors" and those who remained buffered ($pH$ 5.0 or greater) "nonsecretors." These terms have no connotation other than that they are defined relative to each other. The importance of this differentiation in terms of susceptibility to cholera is presented in Table V.

Though the numbers are small, attack in the secretor groups were less than in those individuals with a prolonged buffering effect. The increasing attack rate with increasing vibrio dose in the secretor group was also a suggestive trend. That the same vibrio doses induced disease in almost all the nonsecretors implied that low gastric $pH$ was an important defense against induced cholera.

Serological studies indicated that those men with the most severe disease had demonstrable agglutinins and vibriocidal antibody titers in their serum specimens. The volunteers with temporary carrier states failed to develop humoral antibodies. The development of cholera diarrhea was associated with significant increases in titers of vibriocidal and agglutinating antibodies. However, attempts to correlate baseline vibriocidal antibody titers and immunity have failed to give clear-cut differentiation. There was a trend of greater susceptibility to infection when no vibriocidal antibody titer was present. The significance of these vibriocidal antibodies in a population group unexposed to cholera raises some doubt as to their specificity. Perhaps they were a measure of some cross-reacting antibody and therefore have less relevance than vibriocidal antibodies measured in natives of endemic areas. Additional information will be accumulated on this point.

Rechallenge studies have demonstrated a remarkable resistance to a second dose of organisms. Thus homologous strain rechallenge of 13 volunteers recovered from diarrhea or cholera three to 12 months previously resulted in complete immunity. No stool cultures were found to have vibrios. Heterologous strain rechallenge failed to demonstrate complete immunity. Thus two individuals manifesting diarrhea after an Inaba challenge had a similar illness following Ogawa challenge six to nine months later. Two other volunteers developed diarrhea and carrier status on rechallenge whereas the initial challenge caused only carrier states. These data do suggest a possible role for oral living vaccines as a means of preventing cholera.

## DISCUSSION

Dr. John Snow suspected that a living contagion was contained in the foul water pumped into the Broad Street area. His careful studies pinpointed water as a means of spreading cholera. The diagnosis of cholera in his era could be made only on a clinical basis in the severely dehydrated, usually fatal cases. His analysis compared fatal cases per 10,000 population to the source of their water supply. The actual rate of cholera infection was probably 10 or more times the fatal case rate. The majority of exposed individuals develop mild self-limiting diarrhea and a small percentage have an occult intestinal infection. Such individuals can promulgate the disease by their carrier state. Susceptibility to infection is modified by many factors, one of which is the status of the acid milieu of the stomach. We have little knowledge of the incidence of achlorhydria or hypochlorhydria in the 1850's in England. Snow did notice an increased rate of disease in the poor who lived in crowded homes, and he implied that these individuals may have had greater contact with the causative agent. It is interesting to speculate that perhaps these individuals did indeed have poor acid secretion in the stomach and were therefore more susceptible. In recent epidemics it has been noted that an inordinate number of patients developing cholera have had previous gastrectomies. Pierce[4] has recently demonstrated altered gastric acid secretion in patients during acute cholera. This suggests either that the disease has an inhibiting effect on gastric acid secretion or that the disease had selected out those individuals deficient in acid production.

The vivid descriptions in Snow's writings as to the turbidity of water samples from the Broad Street pump and other water sources in London point to the probability that many bacteria were in suspension. The inoculum from the Broad Street pump might well have been $10^6$ or more organisms per cubic centimeter of water. Such a large dose would insure disease even in patients with a normal stomach. Unfortunately Snow was not able to culture the water to isolate vibrios in 1854. If such an experiment could have been done he could have supplied us with significant data on the number of organisms ingested in nature that cause disease in man. It remains to be demonstrated as to whether coliform bacteria in contaminated water can act synergistically with vibrios in enhancing disease. Under these circumstances perhaps less than 100,000 organisms could initiate disease.

Specific measures to control cholera such as effective vaccines are still in preliminary testing phases. Snow's removal of the pump handle appeared to abort the epidemic in 1854. Unfortunately a similar simple means of interrupting the present spread of cholera does not exist. Until we can provide clean water supplies or an effective vaccine to all individuals this interesting disease will persist.

### REFERENCES

1. Snow, J.: On the Mode of Communication of Cholera—1855. In: *Snow on Cholera*. A reprint of two papers by John Snow. New York and London, Hofner, 1965.
2. Koch, R.: Die Conferenz zur Erörterung der Cholerafrage. *Dtsch. med. Wschr. 10:*499, 1884.
3. Sack, R. B. and Carpenter, C. C. J.: Experimental canine cholera I. Development of the Model. *J. Infect. Dis. 119:* 138-149, 1969.
4. Pierce, N., Hennessey, G. and Mitra, R.: Gastric acidity in cholera. *Clin. Res. 19:* 400, 1971. Abstract.

# CHOLERA: DIAGNOSIS AND TREATMENT*

## CHARLES C. J. CARPENTER, M.D.

Professor of Medicine
Johns Hopkins Medical School
Baltimore, Md.

CHOLERA is an acute illness caused by an enterotoxin elaborated by *Vibrio cholerae* which have colonized the small bowel of a susceptible individual. In its most severe form there is rapid loss of fluid and electrolyte from the gastrointestinal tract, resulting in hypovolemic shock, metabolic acidosis and, if untreated, death.[1]

The clinical onset of cholera is generally that of abrupt, painless, watery diarrhea. In severe cases, several liters of fluid may be lost within a few hours, leading rapidly to profound shock. At varying intervals after onset of diarrhea, vomiting may ensue. This is characteristically effortless and is not preceded by nausea. In the more severe cases, muscle cramps are almost invariably present and commonly involve the calves.

When first seen by the physician, the patient who is severely ill with cholera is cyanotic, has sunken eyes and cheeks, a scaphoid abdomen, poor skin turgor, and thready or absent peripheral pulses. The voice is high-pitched or inaudible; the vital signs include tachycardia, tachypnea, and low or unobtainable blood pressure. There may be either low-grade fever or slight hypothermia. The heart sounds are distant, often inaudible, and bowel sounds are usually hypoactive. Major alterations in mental status are not common in adults; the adult cholera patient usually remains oriented, although apathetic, even in the face of severe hypovolemic shock. Central nervous system abnormalities, ranging from stupor to convulsions and coma, are much more common in pediatric patients, and may occur in up to 10% of small children with cholera. In all epidemics there are large numbers of mild cases in which loss of fluid from the gut is not severe enough to require hospitalization. There are even larger numbers of completely asymptomatic people who transiently excrete *V. cholerae*.[2]

---

*Presented as part of a *Symposium on Cholera* sponsored by The Tropical Disease Center, St. Clare's Hospital, New York, N. Y., and The Merck Company Foundation, Rahway, N. J., held at the Center, June 5, 1971.

In the absence of antimicrobial therapy the gastrointestinal loss of fluid and electrolytes may continue for up to seven days, and subsequent manifestations depend upon the adequacy of replacement therapy. With prompt repletion of fluid and electrolyte, physiologic recovery is remarkably rapid and uniform despite continuing voluminous diarrhea.[1] If therapy is inadequate, the mortality rate in hospitalized cases may exceed 50%. The important causes of death are hypovolemic shock, uncompensated metabolic acidosis, and uremia.

### Diagnosis

In cholera endemic or epidemic areas *the working diagnosis of cholera should be made on the basis of the clinical picture* of severe saline depletion in a patient with a history of abrupt onset of watery and generally painless diarrhea. Therapy should be initiated immediately on the basis of the clinical diagnosis. It is very important to recognize the fact that, although a choleralike illness may be caused by microorganisms other than *V. cholerae*, the resulting physiologic and metabolic abnormalities are essentially the same, so that identical therapy is indicated in all such cases.[3]

Diagnostic culture techniques are relatively simple. A reliable and practical method consists of direct plating of feces on TCBS agar. Typical opaque yellow colonies appear in 18 hours. Final identification requires agglutination with group and type-specific antisera and demonstration of characteristic biochemical reactions. Rapid, tentative diagnosis may be made by direct observation of the characteristic rapid motility of the comma-shaped bacilli in fresh feces by dark-field microscopy. Group and type-specific antisera will immobilize homologous strains and clearly distinguish them from other vibrios.[4]

### Management

#### Intravenous Fluid Therapy

Successful therapy of cholera and the choleralike diarrheal illnesses requires only prompt and adequate replacement of the fluid and electrolytes which have been lost from the gastrointestinal tract.[5] Several interrelated factors are critical to appropriate replacement of these losses of electrolyte fluid. These include the solute concentrations of the fluid used to replace these losses, the route of administration of the replace-

TABLE I. STOOL VOLUME AND ELECTROLYTE PATTERN IN 38 ADULT
CHOLERA PATIENTS DURING FIRST DAY OF TREATMENT

| Mean values $\pm$ S. D. | |
|---|---|
| Volume (l./24 hrs.) | 6.6 $\pm$ 3.1 |
| Sodium (mEq./l.) | 126 $\pm$ 9 |
| Potassium (mEq./l.) | 19 $\pm$ 9 |
| Bicarbonate (mEq./l.) | 47 $\pm$ 10 |

ment fluids, and the rate at which the replacement fluids should be administered.

*Adults.* Table I shows typical stool electrolytes in the severely ill adult cholera patient. The stool is nearly isotonic with plasma, the bicarbonate concentration is roughly twice that of normal plasma, and the potassium concentration is nearly five times that of plasma. The patient who loses this fluid therefore develops an isotonic extracellular fluid deficit and metabolic acidosis, and may develop a clinically significant degree of hypokalemia.

The potassium concentration in the stool varies inversely with the rate of fluid loss, and the figures shown in Table I represent values obtained at a time when the mean stool output was 15% of body weight per 24 hours. With stooling rates of less than 5% of body weight per 24 hours, the stool potassium concentration may be as high as 40 mEq./l., but the absolute loss of potassium with acute diarrheal disease of such magnitude is not great enough to be of major clinical significance. Replacement of fluid in adults should therefore be designed roughly to replace the electrolytes outlined in Table I. In the treatment of the adult patient, there is a fair amount of leeway which will be discussed below.

Based on the known gastrointestinal electrolyte losses, the ideal replacement solution in the adult cholera patient should be roughly isotonic with plasma, with a sodium concentration nearly equal to that in plasma, and a bicarbonate concentration twice that of plasma. When replacement is by the intravenous route a concentration of potassium of 8 to 10 mEq./l. is usually employed, because of the danger of hyperkalemia if fluids with higher potassium concentrations are infused at the rates sometimes required for treatment of the seriously saline-depleted individual. In actual fact, intravenous potassium therapy is seldom *essential* in the adult patient. There are two reasons for this. First, symptomatic

TABLE II. BLOOD CHEMICAL FINDINGS IN 38 CONSECUTIVE CHOLERA
PATIENTS TREATED BY THE 2:1 SALINE:LACTATE REGIMEN

| Mean values ± S. D. | | |
|---|---|---|
| | On admission | Four hours after admission |
| Arterial blood pH | 7.17 ± 0.06 | 7.40 ± 0.05 |
| Plasma bicarbonate (mEq./l.) | 7 ± 4 | 20 ± 3 |
| Plasma potassium (mEq./l.) | 5.6 ± 0.4 | 3.2 ± 0.3 |
| Total plasma protein (gm. %) | 14.2 ± 0.8 | 7.5 ± 0.6 |

TABLE III. INTRAVENOUS FLUIDS FOR CHOLERA:
"5:4:1" SOLUTION FOR ADULTS

| Milliequivalents per liter | |
|---|---|
| Sodium | 133 |
| Chloride | 98 |
| Potassium | 13 |
| Bicarbonate | 48 |

hypokalemia is rarely seen in adults with acute diarrheal disease, despite relatively large potassium losses. Second, absorption of potassium by the small bowel is not significantly impaired during cholera, and repletion of potassium can be achieved effectively by the oral route. In actual fact, 100% recovery of adult patients severely ill with cholera has been achieved by the simple intravenous administration of an isotonic intravenous solution containing two parts sodium chloride to one part sodium lactate.[1] The left column in Table II shows the mean admission blood chemical determinations on 38 consecutive hypotensive, adult cholera patients. Observe the striking elevation in plasma protein concentration, reflecting the loss of roughly half the extracellular fluid volume, and the marked metabolic acidosis. The right column of Table II shows the same values four hours later, after administration of the 2:1 saline: lactate mixture in amounts equal to 10% of the body weight of the patients. Observe that the mean plasma protein concentration and arterial blood pH are now within normal limits, and that, concomitant with extracellular fluid volume expansion and correction of the acidosis, the plasma potassium level has fallen sharply.

A more ideal adult replacement solution, outlined in Table III, can

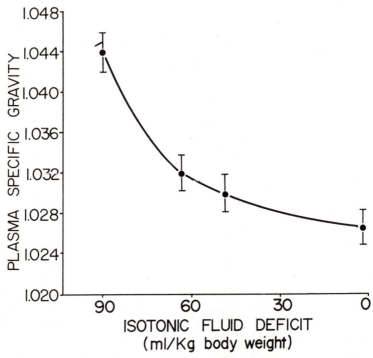

Fig. 1. The relation of plasma specific gravity to isotonic-fluid deficit during the first four hours of treatment of the acute cholera patient. Note that the initial 27 ml./kg. of isotonic fluid repletion caused a greater drop in specific gravity than the subsequent 63 ml./kg. of isotonic fluid repletion. Brackets indicate 95% confidence limits of mean values in 38 consecutive patients.

be prepared by the simple addition of 5 gm. sodium chloride, 4 gm. sodium bicarbonate, and 1 gm. potassium chloride to 1 l. of sterile, pyrogen-free distilled water.[5] In the preparation of this solution the sodium bicarbonate must be added *after* the bottle is autoclaved. Even this relatively simple problem can be overcome by substituting equimolar amounts of sodium acetate, which readily stands autoclaving, for the sodium bicarbonate. The acetate, like the lactate, is rapidly metabolized after intravenous administration, yielding 1 mole of bicarbonate for each mole of acetate which is administered.[6]

The *rate* of intravenous fluid administration is determined by the

TABLE IV. MEAN ELECTROLYTE VALUES IN PEDIATRIC CHOLERA STOOL

| Milliequivalents per liter | |
|---|---|
| Sodium | 98 |
| Chloride | 79 |
| Potassium | 27 |
| Bicarbonate | 32 |

degree of saline depletion. In hypotensive adult patients the initial infusion is given rapidly (at rates of 50 to 100 ml./min.) until a strong radial pulse has been restored. Subsequently the fluids are infused in quantities equal to the gastrointestinal losses. Ideally, each patient should be placed on a "cholera cot," with the buttocks positioned over a hole leading directly to a collecting bucket. If the fluid losses cannot be accurately measured (i.e., if cholera cots and calibrated buckets are not available), intravenous fluids should be given at a rate sufficient to maintain a normal radial pulse volume and normal skin turgor.[7] Overhydration can be avoided by careful observation of the neck veins and auscultation of the lungs. Close observation of the patient is mandatory during the first two days of therapy; an adult patient can lose up to 1 l. of isotonic fluid per hour during the first 24 hours of illness.

Although determination of whole blood or plasma specific-gravity has been employed historically as a means to estimate fluid deficit in cholera patients, this technique has been found in recent years to be of less value under epidemic conditions than the careful, sequential clinical evaluation of the patient. This specific gravity technique has several important limitations. 1) This test, like any other, is subject to errors in sampling, handling, and reading which are likely to be multiplied during epidemic situations. 2) The correlation between isotonic fluid deficit and plasma specific gravity is *not* a straight-line one, as demonstrated by Figure 1, and the technique therefore fails to provide a consistently accurate means of determining requirements of fluid. 3) It is further my strong impression that, in the management of large numbers of cholera patients, emphasis on any technique other than bedside evaluation tends to detract from the quality of the care of patients.

The *route* of intravenous fluid infusion is generally no great problem in adult patients, in whom a needle of large bore, No. 16 or No. 18, can generally be inserted in an antecubital vein.

Table V. INTRAVENOUS FLUIDS FOR CHOLERA:
PEDIATRIC CHOLERA SOLUTION

| | |
|---|---|
| Sodium (mEq./l.) | 94 |
| Chloride (m.Eq./l.) | 64 |
| Potassium (mEq./l.) | 15 |
| Acetate (mEq./l.) | 45 |
| Glucose (gm.%) | 2 |

*Children.* The stool-electrolyte pattern in children, shown in Table IV, varies significantly from that of the adult in that the mean sodium concentration is significantly lower, and the mean potassium concentration is significantly higher than that in adult patients.[8] The basis for these differences is not yet understood, but they are of critical importance in determining the optimal therapeutic regimen for patients weighing less than 20 kg.

The pediatric patient not only requires a different intravenous solution because of the different composition of the stool, but the patient also requires a more precise correction of the electrolyte losses. Table V shows the composition of fluid which appears appropriate for the treatment of pediatric diarrhea.[9] This regimen, developed by the U.S. Naval Medical Research Unit in Manila, takes into consideration the hypotonicity of the pediatric stool losses, the relatively greater potassium requirements, and the fact that serious hypoglycemia not uncommonly accompanies severe diarrhea in pediatric patients.[10] There is less leeway in pediatric than in adult patients, both in regard to the tonicity and in regard to the potassium concentration of the administered fluids. Whereas the adult rarely develops serious problems—albeit he gets very thirsty—with moderate degrees of hypernatremia, the pediatric patient may develop organic brain damage when the serum sodium concentration is in the 160 to 170 mEq./l. range. The intravenous administration of an isotonic solution to a pediatric patient with diarrheal disease may therefore cause serious brain damage or death, *unless* appropriate amounts of water are given by mouth.[8] The latter is sometimes difficult to achieve under epidemic conditions, and it is therefore advisable that intravenous replacement solutions for pediatric cholera be significantly hypotonic with respect to plasma.

By the same token the pediatric cholera patient not only loses relatively more potassium than his adult counterpart, because of the greater potassium concentration in the stool, but is also at greater risk from complications of hypokalemia. These complications may include paralytic ileus, hypotension, and cardiac arrhythmias which are sometimes fatal. It is therefore critical that pediatric intravenous replacement fluids contain potassium in roughly the amounts indicated in Table V.[11]

Replacement of electrolyte losses is more difficult in the pediatric patient; it depends on an accurate clinical evaluation of the initial isotonic fluid deficit. Determination of the body weight on admission is most helpful. The following guidelines are then useful.[12] *Mild dehydration* (slightly decreased skin turgor and tachycardia, but good peripheral pulses and normal sensorium) indicates an isotonic-fluid deficit of about 5% of body weight. *Moderate dehydration* (marked decrease in skin turgor, tachycardia, and hypotension, but normal sensorium) indicates a fluid deficit of 6 to 8% of body weight. *Severe dehydration* (above signs plus cyanosis, stupor or coma, absent peripheral pulses) indicates a fluid deficit of 10 to 12% of body weight. Approximately one half the initial estimated fluid deficit should be administered during the first hour of treatment, and the remaining half should be given during the next two to three hours of therapy, with frequent evaluation of the pulse, neck veins, and lungs in order to prevent over- or underhydration. Following initial rehydration the rate of intravenous fluid administration should be determined by the rate of gastrointestinal fluid loss. Ideally, as in the adult, this should be ascertained by placing the child on a cholera cot and directly measuring the fluid losses. If, however, cholera cots are not available, frequent assessment of clinical parameters of hydration are entirely satisfactory for the determination of fluid requirements. Continuing clinical evaluation is, in fact, essential even when losses of fluid can be determined accurately.

Finding and maintaining an adequate *route* for intravenous fluid therapy is frequently a critical problem in children, in whom successful therapy is absolutely dependent upon the ability of skilled personnel to find and secure a good vein. Seriously saline-depleted children often have collapsed peripheral veins, but the external jugular vein is generally visible after compression at the base of the neck. Occasionally the femoral vein must be used initially to infuse fluids until other veins become apparent. Pediatric scalp-vein needles are most helpful for maintenance of intravenous fluid infusions in the smaller patients.

TABLE VI. EFFECT OF TETRACYCLINE ON STOOL VOLUME IN
CHOLERA PATIENTS, 1963 STUDY

| | Mean values ± S. D. | | |
| | Tetracycline (10 patients) | No tetracycline (10 patients) | P value by "t" test |
|---|---|---|---|
| Stool volume (liters) | | | |
| Day 1 | 6.6 ± 2.1 | 8.3 ± 3.3 | $P > 0.3$ |
| Day 2 | 2.2 ± 1.6 | 4.3 ± 3.1 | $P > 0.05$ |
| Day 3 | 0.9 ± 1.0 | 5.0 ± 4.1 | $P < 0.01$ |
| Day 4 | 0.4 ± 1.1 | 3.8 ± 3.4 | $P < 0.01$ |
| Totals | 10.6 ± 4.9 | 24.0 ± 17.8 | $P < 0.05$ |

## ANTIMICROBIAL THERAPY

Although intravenous fluid therapy, when promptly and adequately administered, results in survival of virtually all cholera patients, the intravenous fluid requirements may be staggering, and occasional patients have required intravenous fluids in amounts equal to twice their body weight. In fact, the *average* intravenous fluid requirement in one carefully studied group of adult cholera patients was 24 l. The logistic problems presented by such fluid requirements are overwhelming in the impoverished rural areas in which cholera outbreaks most frequently occur. It was therefore a welcome finding, in 1963, that tetracycline therapy results in a 60% reduction in gastrointestinal fluid loss (Table VI), and an equally great reduction in duration of diarrhea in the seriously ill cholera patient.[13] Tetracycline, in the dosage of 40 mg./kg. per day, given in divided doses for two days, also eliminates *V. cholerae* from the stool in the great majority of cholera patients. Other antimicrobial agents, most notably furazolidone and chloramphenicol, have also proved highly effective in reducing gastrointestinal fluid losses in cholera, but both these agents appear to be slightly less effective than tetracycline.

Tetracycline therapy has therefore more than doubled the number of patients who can be treated adequately with a given amount of intravenous fluids. Since the availability of intravenous fluids is frequently the limiting factor in dealing with outbreaks of cholera, antimicrobial therapy has proved to be a major advance in the management of cholera. Even with appropriate antimicrobial therapy, however, the

TABLE VII. COMPOSITION OF ORAL GLUCOSE-ELECTROLYTE SOLUTION

| | |
|---|---|
| Sodium | 100 mEq./l. |
| Potassium | 10 mEq./l. |
| Chloride | 70 mEq./l. |
| Bicarbonate | 40 mEq./l. |
| Glucose | 120 mM./l. |
| Osmolarity | 327 mOsm./l. |

requirements of fluid remain large. The *average* intravenous fluid requirement in this group of tetracycline-treated patients shown in Table VI was still 10 l.

## ORAL ELECTROLYTE THERAPY

The development of oral therapy for cholera in the late 1960's was, therefore, another milestone in the treatment of this disease, as it further extended by several fold the number of patients to whom adequate treatment could be given in situations in which the supply of intravenous fluids is limited. The development of oral therapy is a particularly interesting one, as it involves the direct clinical extension of an observation which had previously appeared to be relevant only in the realm of basic physiologic research: namely, that intraluminal glucose enhances absorption of sodium by the mammalian small intestine. As expressed earlier in this symposium, the primary problem in cholera is that of the increased *secretion* of isotonic fluid by the small intestine caused by the cholera enterotoxin. The enterotoxin has no significant effect on movement of sugar from gut lumen to plasma. Nor does the enterotoxin alter the enhancement of lumen-to-plasma movement of sodium which is caused by intraluminal glucose. It has therefore been possible to develop a solution containing both glucose and sodium which, when administered orally to the actively purging cholera patient, can maintain adequate fluid and electrolyte balance.[14, 15] Such a solution is presented in Table VII. Although solutions with a wide variety of glucose concentrations, as well as certain variations in electrolyte concentrations, have been tested under field conditions, solutions approximating that shown in this table have proved most successful in maintaining fluid balance in both pediatric and adult cholera patients. While all severely saline-depleted cholera patients require intravenous fluids until adequate circulation is restored, the oral route has been used successfully *both* for maintenance therapy in the more severely ill patients *and* for the entire

245

course of therapy in patients with less severe disease. Although oral therapy has been of greatest value in adults, it can also be effectively employed in children who are alert and able to retain orally administered solutions.[16] It is important to emphasize that successful management of the cholera patient with oral therapy demands just as close supervision, with careful monitoring of pulse volume, skin turgor, and neck veins, as does management with intravenous solutions. Supplemental intravenous fluids must be administered whenever clinical signs of saline depletion recur.

Of critical importance to the proper management of the cholera patient is the knowledge that hypotension, when present, is entirely due to hypovolemia. A number of pharmacologic agents, including cardiotonic drugs, sympathomimetic amines, central nervous system stimulants, steroids and antiperistaltic agents have sometimes been employed in the treatment of this disease. The use of all such agents is strongly contraindicated. Certain of these agents are clearly harmful (e.g., by precipitating cardiac arrhythmias or intensifying renal ischemia in the hypotensive patient), and the use of any such agents detracts from the primary goal of prompt and adequate fluid and electrolyte replacement.

### New Therapeutic Approaches

The essence of this discussion has been that every cholera patient should survive if he receives adequate replacement therapy. Adequate therapy for patients in cholera endemic areas has often been, and frequently still is, impossible because of the lack of adequate supplies of sterile, pyrogen-free fluids. The requirement for such fluids has been greatly decreased, first by the use of appropriate antimicrobial therapy and, more recently, by the use of an oral electrolyte replacement regimen. Patients still, however, die of cholera, and the mortality rates in certain of the recent outbreaks in Africa have been extremely high. Even with adjuvant antimicrobial therapy and oral electrolyte replacement, adequate intravenous fluids have often not been available in the areas in which cholera has occurred. The recent advances in our understanding of the mechanism by which the cholera enterotoxin acts has led to the hope of developing an agent which, without causing unacceptable side effects, will rapidly reverse the action of the cholera enterotoxin. Since the enterotoxin appears to achieve its effect by stimulating adenyl cyclase in the gut epithelial cell wall,[17, 18] it is hoped that enterotoxin

246

action may be blocked either by an antagonist of adenyl cyclase or by an agent which lowers intracellular levels of cyclic $3'5'$ adenosine monophosphate. Considerable research is presently being directed toward this goal.

## REFERENCES

1. Carpenter, C. C. J., Mondal, A., Sack, R. B., Mitra, P. P., Dans, P. E., Wells, S. A., Hinman, E. J. and Chaudhuri, R. N.: Clinical studies in Asiatic cholera. II. *Bull. Hopkins Hosp. 118*:174, 1966.
2. Mosley, W. H.: The role of immunity in cholera. A review of epidemiological and serological studies. *Texas Rep. Biol. Med. 27*:227, 1969.
3. Lindenbaum, J., Greenough, W. B., Benenson, A. S., Oseasohn, R., Rizvi, S. and Saad, A.: Non-vibrio cholera. *Lancet 1*:1081, 1965.
4. Benenson, A. S., Islam, M. R. and Greenough, W. B.: Rapid identification of *Vibrio cholerae* by darkfield microscopy. *Bull. WHO 30*:827, 1964.
5. Gordon, R. S., Feeley, J. C., Greenough, W. B., Sprinz, H. and Oseasohn, R. O.: Cholera. Combined staff clinic conference at the National Institutes of Health. *Ann. Intern. Med. 64*:1288, 1966.
6. Watten, R. H., Gutman, R. A. and Fresh, J. W.: Comparison of acetate, lactate and bicarbonate in treatment of the acidosis of cholera. *Lancet 2*:512, 1969.
7. Carpenter, C. C. J., Mitra, P. P., Sack, R. B., Wells, S. A., Dans, P. E. and Chaudhuri, R. N.: Clinical evaluation of fluid requirements in Asiatic cholera. *Lancet 1*:726, 1965.
8. Griffith, L. S. C., Fresh, J. W., Watten, R. H. and Villaroman, M. P.: Electrolyte replacement in pediatric cholera. *Lancet 1*:1197, 1967.
9. Gutman, R. H., Drutz, D. J., Whalen, G. E. and Watten, R. H. Double blind fluid therapy evaluation in pediatric cholera. *Pediatrics 44*:922, 1969.
10. Hirschhorn, N., Lindenbaum, J., Greenough, W. B. and Alam, S. M.: Hypo-

glycemia in children with acute diarrhea. *Lancet 2*:128, 1966.
11. Lindenbaum, J., Akbar, R., Gordon, R. S., Greenough, W. B. and Islam, W. R. Cholera in children. *Lancet 1*:1066, 1966.
12. Mahalanobis, D., Wallace, C. K., Kallen, R. J., Mondal, A. and Pierce, N. F.: Water and electrolyte losses due to cholera in infants and small children: A recovery balance study. *Pediatrics 44*:374, 1970.
13. Wallace, C. K., Anderson, P. N., Brown, T. C., Khanra, S. R., Lewis, G. W., Pierce, N. F., Sanyal, S. N., Segre, G. V. and Waldman, R. H.: Optimal antibiotic therapy in cholera. *Bull. WHO 39*:239, 1968.
14. Hirschhorn, N., Kinzie, J. L., Sachar, D. B., Northrup, R. S., Taylor, J. O., Ahmad, Z. and Phillips, R. A.: Decrease in net stool output in cholera during intestinal perfusion with glucose-containing solutions. *New Eng. J. Med. 279*:176, 1968.
15. Pierce, N. F., Sack, R. B., Mitra, R. C., Banwell, J. G., Brigham, K. L., Fedson, D. S. and Mondal, A.: Replacement of water and electrolyte losses in cholera by an oral glucose-electrolyte solution. *Ann. Intern. Med. 70*:1173, 1969.
16. Nalin, D. R. and Cash, R. A.: Oral or nasogastric maintenance in pediatric cholera patients. *J. Pediat. 78*:355, 1971.
17. Kimberg, D., Field, M., Johnson, J., Henderson, A. and Gershan, E.: Stimulation of intestinal mucosal adenyl cyclase by cholera enterotoxin and prostaglandins. *J. Clin. Invest. 50*:1218, 1971.
18. Sharp, G. W. G. and Hynie, S.: Stimulation of intestinal adenyl cyclase by cholera toxin. *Nature 229*:266, 1971.

247

# THE CONTROL OF CHOLERA*

ABRAM S. BENENSON, M.D.

Professor and Chairman
Department of Community Medicine
University of Kentucky
Lexington, Kentucky

WHEN, like the Huns of old, cholera swept from Asia into Europe, it wreaked havoc indeed. As it spread into Russia in 1830, 10% or more of the population of cities might die within a few weeks, often literally within hours after onset. Since it affected principally the poor and the destitute, many considered it a divine and just punishment. Unfortunately appropriate prayers to control the epidemic were not discovered. A more pragmatic Russian government established quarantines around infected communities, hoping by physical restraint to check the spread of the disease. Despite rigorous enforcement with floggings and executions, this measure also failed. A situation developed which was described by a contemporary Russian writer thus: "What is remarkable is the terror which the cholera inspires among people who count the plague as nothing. From the first noble to the last slave . . . all flee the sick and abandon them to their own devices. All natural bonds disappear, and as honor no longer exists, egoism appears in all its nakedness, in all its horror."[1] The military cordon failed before these pressures, and even the double cordon established around Vienna did not prevent the entry of cholera in 1831.

The medical profession was as confused by cholera as the lay public. Unlike smallpox, the chain of infection was not obvious, so that a great dispute ensued whether the disease was contagious or not. The resemblance of the cholera case to arsenic poisoning was recognized, and indeed rumors spread several times that this disease was in fact a mass poisoning of the common people by the nobility or, on occasion, by the medical profession. In the ensuing riots, the police and governmental officials were attacked. On at least one occasion, physicians were slaughtered, and the sick were removed from the cholera hospitals to save

---

*Presented as part of a *Symposium on Cholera* sponsored by The Tropical Disease Center, St. Clare's Hospital, New York, N. Y., and The Merck Company Foundation, Rahway, N. J., held at the Center, June 5, 1971.

them from the black magic presumed to be practiced by the doctors. It took the careful studies of John Snow in 1849 to 1855 to introduce the first pertinent glimmer of sense.[2] Logical analysis of carefully collected data on mortality led this anesthesiologist to the hypothesis that cholera evacuations were being mixed with water used for drinking and that this caused the disease. Snow tested his hypothesis by comparing the incidence of cholera in the customers of two different water companies. He was able to demonstrate that the mortality rates were 14 times higher among those using unfiltered Thames River water than among those whose water came from a better source. His dramatic removal of the handle of the Broad Street pump was a logical direct action. The subsequent absence of new cases is usually attributed to this act; the modern day epidemiologist is more impressed by the fortunate timing since the epidemic had already exhausted the supply of susceptibles.

Despite this understanding of the spread of disease, pandemics recurred again and again to run their natural course. In 1883 Robert Koch isolated the etiological organism and, within a year, J. Ferrán introduced immunization against cholera. Ferrán injected 1 ml. doses of living culture of the organisms; the severe reactions, sometimes including death, were felt justified in the face of so catastrophic a disease. Unfortunately adequate proof that it was protective could not be developed. Subsequent studies with different vaccines, including a living attentuated vaccine prepared by Waldemar M. Haffkine as well as killed vaccines, have indicated varying degrees of protectiveness. While some of the studies were well-designed, others had defects so that there was doubt whether the vaccine protected against cholera.[3]

International sanitary conferences in Constantinople in 1866 and in Vienna in 1874 established the concept of international quarantine and quarantine stations. The measures for international control of cholera in the 1960's were based on these facts and observations. A traveler who had been immunized within a six-month period could come from an infected area and move freely throughout the world, although surveillance might be maintained for five days. Improved sanitation was advocated; indeed cholera gave great impetus to the establishment of safe supplies of drinking water. In fact, the epidemic of 1832 is credited with being the force which established the Croton Aqueduct as the source of potable water for the City of New York; this source replaced a supply used only by those who could not afford to have water brought into the city in hogsheads from "pure" springs and wells in the countryside.[4]

The studies carried out over the past 10 years have provided much information on which to develop a more logical set of control measures. For once, studies were under way before the epidemic hit, a circumstance for which credit must be given not to the foresight of a bacteriologist, but to that of an eminent authority in the field of rickettsiae and viruses, the late Joseph E. Smadel.

Properly designed and adequately controlled field studies have been carried out that have tested the efficacy of various cholera vaccines in Pakistan,[5, 6] India,[7] and the Philippines.[8] Whole cell vaccines and purified derivatives produced a significant reduction in the incidence of clinical disease, with 50 to 90% fewer cases than occurred in comparable groups who received a control vaccine (typhoid vaccine or tetanus toxoid). Unfortunately this protection lasted for only a short time, so that the vaccine must be given within a few months before exposure to disease is expected if it is to be protective. Further, difficulty is encountered in carrying out the immunization program. Those who volunteer for vaccination are usually the better-educated members of higher social levels who very rarely develop cholera. Those under the greatest risk of acquiring cholera are those who are most reluctant to accept the vaccine; great effort and expense is required to find and protect those who need it!

Field studies have clearly demonstrated that the classical dehydrated cholera patient represents the peak of the iceberg with many, many more asymptomatic cases or cases with simple diarrhea.[9, 10] The vaccine studies have shown that while vaccination does reduce the incidence of manifest disease, no clear reduction in the number of carriers can be assumed.[5] Clinical studies have shown that a carrier state can persist for prolonged periods of time,[11] and that this carrier state can persist as a biliary infection with negative stools and rectal swabs, so that infection can be demonstrated only by culturing duodenal aspirates or saline purge fluid.[12]

Failure of quarantine measures was predicted 100 years ago on the basis that those most likely to carry the organism would probably not be so considerate as to report to quarantine stations. Experience has borne this out in that many introductions of disease into clean areas

CONTROL OF CHOLERA IN THE 1970's

1) Effective treatment of cholera as a diarrheal case.
2) Bacteriological surveillance of diarrheal diseases.
3) Chemoprophylaxis for members of the patient's hearth-group.
4) Sanitary improvements:
    Water supply.
    Disposal of excreta.
5) Health education.
6) Immunizations on a voluntary basis.
7) Elimination of quarantine measures.

have been attributed to smugglers, fishermen, or others who cross borders at undesignated points. Among those who do properly pass through the quarantine station, vaccine will not assure that the traveler is not a carrier and it will not guarantee that the individual may not develop clinical disease. Even when excessive measures have been applied by some countries, a rectal swab and a requirement for a negative culture will not detect the individuals whose gall bladders and duodena contain cholera vibrios which, under appropriate conditions, can transit the intestinal tract.

What, then, is the appropriate control program for the 1970's? I give first priority to the implementation of the very effective treatment now available (see accompanying table). The treatment of cholera is that of any dehydrating diarrhea regardless of etiological organism. The countries where cholera is most likely to occur are those in which diarrhea is a common disease; dehydrating diarrheas not associated with infection from *Vibrio cholerae* occur frequently. Intravenous rehydration fluid must be available without delay where and when the case may occur. This will be so only when cases of diarrheal disease are treated as though they had cholera; this will establish and maintain skill in the practitioners; it will also assure a flow of supplies for intravenous and oral therapy to the places of need. When the public knows how effective cholera treatment can be, panic is allayed, confidence is generated, and the cooperation of the population is insured. In his report to the Executive Board of WHO, Dr. Marcelino G. Candau, director-general, stated in January 1971 that "Today, cholera is one of the most rewarding diseases to treat; no patient with uncomplicated cholera arriving at the treatment center with his heart beating should

251

die. A moribund case of cholera given proper intravenous rehydration should be quite comfortable in a few hours time, and recovery is complete with no sequellae." [13]

When cholera does enter a country the requirement for treatment materials and facilities will be sharply increased. This can be anticipated by early recognition that cholera vibrios are present in the population. This is best achieved by establishing adequate laboratory facilities for routine bacteriological surveillance of diarrhea cases. Only simple bacteriological techniques are involved. If the El Tor biotype is involved, culturing sewage may give early warning. [14]

When cholera is recognized in an individual, 10 to 20% of hearth-group contacts will be infected; some may develop disease while the others may spread the organisms. [15] The administration of 1 gm. of tetracycline daily for five days will free these individuals of infection, preventing secondary cases or spread of disease. [16]

The ultimate control of cholera rests in the development of a level of sanitation which will avoid fecal-oral transmission of the causal organism. Disease persists in areas of overcrowding and poor sanitation. The provision of a safe potable water supply and the establishment of techniques for safe excreta disposal provide better areas for investment of the time, effort, and money rather than dissipating these scarce resources in any immunization program. The part played by food, [17] whether contaminated by polluted water or by poor hygienic practices indicates the need for appropriate health education.

Immunization, shown to reduce significantly the risk to the individual, must be made available for those who desire it; but in the control of cholera in the community it plays a relatively minor role.

Many are now concerned about overpopulation and express concern that our preventive measures aggravate the problem. This is not a new concern; Brigham, [18] in 1832 published *A Treatise on Epidemic Cholera*, in which he states that in 1823:

> In China, the ravages of the cholera were also great, in consequences of the numerous canals, and the immense population of the country. The Russian authorities urged the Mandarins to arrest the disease by adopting some preventive or preservative measures. But they were told in answer, that the malady would give more space in the world to those who survived it, and besides, that the cholera chose its victims from

among the filthy and the intemperate, and that no person of courage who lived with moderation and surrounded by cleanliness, would die of the disease.

We hope to achieve the cleanliness and must depend on family planning programs to provide the living space.

Here in the dispassionate atmosphere of a well-sanitated city which has had no case of cholera near it for more than 60 years we can draw up a modern control program, but outdated practices are still extant. Five years ago, a military cordon was established through the middle of Iran, preventing westward movement of anyone until chloramphenicol had been taken for three days. Within the year, a quarantine on travel was imposed in an area of a country where cholera appeared, resulting in dislocated persons with inadequate facilities. Some countries have denied the presence of the disease which was present, and others have imposed varying restrictive measures. To quote from the WHO Expert Committee on Cholera in 1967: "If, instead of taking excessive, ineffective and outdated measures, countries were to fight cholera in a spirit of international cooperation and in the light of modern scientific achievement, many lives and resources can be saved."[19] The United States has taken a positive lead in this direction by eliminating the requirement for cholera vaccination for travelers coming to this country from cholera-infected areas. In his statement, Dr. Jesse L. Steinfeld, Surgeon General of the U. S. Public Health Service, stated, "There is clear evidence that cholera vaccine is of little use in preventing the spread of cholera across borders. We have today excellent treatment for cholera; the only effective method for preventing the spread of disease is improvement of environmental sanitation."[20] The retention of the concept of quarantinability of this disease maintains the tendency to apply restrictive measures, even though they are admittedly ineffectual, and to foster nonreporting for fear that repressive measures will be applied against the reporting country with loss of trade or tourism.

In this country, if cholera should be imported, it would be no more than another case of diarrheal disease with strictly limited, if any, spread. With international cooperation and improvement of levels of sanitation and the standard of living, it is hoped that this will soon apply worldwide.

## REFERENCES

1. McGrew, R. E.: *Russia and the Cholera 1823-1832*. Madison and Milwaukee, Univ. Wisconsin Press, 1965, p. 11.
2. Snow, J.: *On the Mode of Communication of Cholera*. London, Churchill, 1855.
3. Cvjetanovic, B.: Earlier Field Studies of the Effectiveness of Cholera Vaccines. In: *Proc. Cholera Res. Symp.* 355-61, 1965.
4. Rosenberg, C. E.: *The Cholera Years. The United States in 1832, 1849 and 1866*. Chicago, Univ. Chicago Press, 1962, p. 103.
5. Benenson, A. S., Mosley, W. H., Fahimuddin, M and Oseasohn, R. O.: Cholera vaccine field trials in East Pakistan. 2. Effectiveness in the field. *Bull. WHO 38*:359-72, 1968.
6. Mosley, W. H.: The role of immunity in cholera. A review of epidemiological and serological studies. *Tex. Rep. Biol. Med. 27*:227-41, 1969.
7. Das Gupta, A. et al.: Controlled field trial of the effectiveness of cholera and cholera El Tor vaccines in Calcutta. *Bull. WHO 37*:371-85, 1967.
8. Azurin, J. C. et al.: A controlled field trial of the effectiveness of cholera and cholera El Tor vaccines in the Philippines. *Bull. WHO 37*:703-27, 1967.
9. Yen, C. H.: A recent study of cholera with reference to an outbreak in Taiwan in 1962. *Bull. WHO 30*:811-25, 1964.
10. McCormack, William M., Shafiqul Islam, M., Fahimuddin, M. and Mosley, Wiley H.: A community study of inapparent cholera infections. *Amer. J. Epidemiol. 89*:658-44, 1969.
11. Azurin, J. C., Kobari, K., Barua, D., Alvero, M., Gomez, C. Z., Dizon, J. J., Nakano, E., Suplido, R. and Ledesma, L.: A long-term carrier of cholera: Cholera Dolores. *Bull. WHO 37*:745-49, 1967.
12. Gangarosa, E. J., Saghari, H., Emile, J. and Siadat, H.: Detection of *vibrio cholerae* biotype El Tor by purging. *Bull. WHO 34*:362-69, 1966.
13. Candau, M. G.: The seventh cholera pandemic. *WHO Chron. 25*:155-59, 1971.
14. Bart, K. J., Khan, M. and Mosley, W. H.: Isolation of *Vibrio cholerae* from nightsoil during epidemics of classical and El Tor cholera in East Pakistan. *Bull. WHO 43*:421-29, 1970.
15. Martin, A. R., Mosley, W. H., Biswas, S., Binapani, A., Shamsa, and Huq, I.: Epidemiologic analysis of endemic cholera in urban East Pakistan. *Amer. J. Epidem. 89*:572-82, 1969.
16. McCormack, W. M., Chowdhury, A. M., Jahangir, N., Fariduddin Ahmed, A. B. and Mosley, W. H.: Tetracycline prophylaxis in families of cholera patients. *Bull. WHO 38*:787-92, 1968.
17. Benenson, A. S., Ahmad, S. Z. and Ostasohn, R. O.: Person-to-person transmission of cholera. *Proceedings of the Cholera Research Symposium,* January 24-29, 1965, Honolulu, Hawaii, and Bethesda, Md.: 332-36, 1965.
18. Brigham, A.: *A Treatise on Epidemic Cholera*. Hartford, Huntington, 1832.
19. WHO Expert Committee on Cholera, Second Report. *WHO Tech. Rep. Series*. No. 352, 1967.
20. Steinfeld, J. *J.A.M.A. 215*:381, 1971.

# RECOLLECTIONS OF CHOLERA AT THE TURN OF THE CENTURY*

VICTOR G. HEISER, M.D.

Former Director of the Far East
Rockefeller Foundation
New York, N. Y.

AFTER hearing from previous speakers of recent experiences with cholera it may be of interest to mention a few experiences in the far distant past.

I did not see cholera until 1903. When I arrived in the Philippines the army was struggling to control an outbreak that had already caused 150,000 deaths. I lived with the army officers who were in charge of the epidemic, so I had a good opportunity to inform myself about cholera. Two years later I was placed in charge of the health of the Philippine Islands, and dealing with cholera became one of my important duties, so the experience I had had with the outbreak dealt with by the army proved very valuable, as it made it unnecessary to try means that they had found would not succeed.

At the beginning of an outbreak the mortality of cholera was often 75% or more but, as the epidemic continued, the mortality declined. After the sixth month the mortality had declined very often to 2%.

Soon after taking charge we had a cable from President Theodore Roosevelt stating that he had a letter from a doctor in Ohio who found that in the 1862 epidemic they used quinine and had a mortality of only 2%. The doctor stated that he had informed us of this marvelous remedy but we had failed to use it. As the president obviously wanted the Ohio doctor's treatment tried, and as I could see no harm in doing so — we had no drug that had any influence on the mortality — we applied the Ohio doctor's quinine treatment to the first five cases who came to the hospital. We sent a cable to the president informing him that we had tried it on five cases and they had all died, and asked if he wished to have the treatment continued.

*Presented as part of a *Symposium on Cholera* sponsored by The Tropical Disease Center, St. Clare's Hospital, New York, N. Y., and The Merck Company Foundation, Rahway, N. J., held at the Center, June 5, 1971.

Never had I believed it possible that an answer would come from Washington so quickly. We had barely filed our cable to the president when an answer came with a big *No*. It was obvious that the Ohio doctor was dealing with cases of cholera that had come down from Quebec and in all probability were in their last stages, or in the 2% mortality rate, so any treatment would have been just as effective as the quinine he was administering.

Cholera often kills with the speed of lightning. One noon, walking on one of the streets of Manila, I saw a man jump into the air and fall down. In the few seconds that it took me to reach him, I found that he was dead. Autopsy and culture showed that he had died of cholera.

On another occasion, I attended an evening lecture with a friend and said good night to him at about 10 p.m., when he left for his apartment. The next morning when I arrived at the office I found a cable from his family instructing us what to do with the body. It seems that soon after reaching his apartment he was stricken and died almost instantly.

On another occasion when I arrived in my office one morning I found there were 15 or 20 cases of cholera reported in widely varying sections of Manila. It did not take us long to learn that people were rowing out into the bay and scooping up fresh water that was bubbling up in the salt water. These people were not only drinking it themselves but were bringing it to their friends, as it was regarded as a miracle. What had actually happened was that a sewer line that extended out into the bay had broken, and fresh water sewage was bubbling up through the salt water.